The Breastfeeding Class You Never Had: Getting Started Nursing Your Baby

By Ann Bennett IBCLC, RLC LLL

DISCLAIMER

My goal in this book is to get the information out there. I don't want anyone to feel the language in this book excludes them from the information. Families come in all varieties. The main thing that makes us all the same is that we are all human, and we all love. Two humans who love a little human. In this book, I use the pronoun he for the baby. I do this to make a distinction between the Mom for whom I use she. I had boys, so for me the baby was always a he. I also use husband, because again, I am writing from my own point of view, and I have a husband. So if your family looks different than this, just sub in your preferred pronoun and title in the spots for he, she, and husband. One of my dear friends has a favorite quote about love: "Love is the most universal, formidable, and mysterious of cosmic energies." by Fr. Teilhard de Chardin SJ. Simply the whole universe and everything in it is created out of and by Love.

Contents

THANKS

The thanks of this book could be pages and pages. From prayer support, to editing help, listening to me read over the phone, cover dimensions, knitting distractions, walks around the block, and self care reminders... I must say I have the best group of friends. THANK YOU! I also want to thank all the Moms in my care who had the biggest struggles. They were not just overcomers and survivors but THEY THRIVED. You inspire me and teach me that it is never too late, and there is always hope! THANK YOU!

DEDICATION

To my children who are still my best teachers, especially my high need baby who increased my prayer life, got me to my very first LLL meeting, and taught me babies have preferences. To my easy baby, who made me feel like I was doing everything right, when in reality, he was just an easy baby. To my husband who has always been my biggest fan, and to the Lord, who is the Giver of my gift of knowledge, and without His help I would not be able to do this. Thank You.
Every Praise.

Introduction
The Breastfeeding Class You Never Had

If you are picking up this book you are either nursing your baby, pregnant and want to nurse your baby, or looking for help for someone who is one of the above.

I am writing this book to try and save you some reinventing of the wheel, to help you understand normal vs. needs attention and mainly to just get the facts out there. I have been an International Board Certified Lactation Consultant for fifteen years. And while I love my job and feel it is why God put me on the planet, I keep saying the same things over and over again, year after year, to Moms and Providers, Dads and Grandmas, like the Groundhog Day movie with a breastfeeding theme. Also, I hear at least once a week, "Why did no one tell me this?"

The "this" could be anything. How long do babies nurse? What is mastitis? What is tongue tie? I had no idea you could tell how much a baby is getting by counting their diapers. The list goes on. Every time someone asks me, "How did I not know this?," I think, "I'm going to write a book."

Then there are the breastfeeding classes I've taught: in homes and in Midwives' offices, over the phone while walking around the neighborhood trying to exercise, for neighbors, and for friends' kids who are now having babies. The overwhelming response is, "Because I took your class, it went great!" Before you think I am a miracle worker, let me clarify: these Moms still had some obstacles, but they knew what the obstacles were, what to do about them, and how to get help.

So that's my promise to you. Reading this book will give you the tools you need to understand what to expect, what is normal and what needs attention. I'm not going to sugar coat it for you, nor am I going to lie to you and say it's always super easy.

But I will tell you I nursed my own two boys, and it is still one of the best times of my life. I didn't say easiest, but I did say best.

So for my future grandchildren and for you: we, along with women for thousands of years, are doing this! Breastfeeding works. If it didn't, I wouldn't be here writing this, and you wouldn't be reading it. If it was just too complicated and painful, Betty Sue cave woman would have said, "This is just too hard." She would have left her baby in the cave alone while she went picking berries with Thelma, and we would have all died out. Mammals nurse. You're a mammal. No matter how challenging it gets remember, at the one year old birthday party you're going to look back at this time, and it's all going to be a blur. I'm rooting for you, pom poms waving, mega phone up! You've got this!

Chapter One:
Why?

It is hard to understand how to do something if you don't understand the "whys" of doing it. A super simple example of this idea is, why would you not grab the pan off the stove without using a potholder? It will burn you. The reasons that we stick with something are usually because we understand there is a benefit of doing it. If you could pick up a hot pan and you did not burn yourself, or if you never had to charge your phone and the battery would last forever then you would never use potholders, or plug in your phone. When times get tough with nursing, it's good to have a reminder of why breastfeeding is so important. To put this in breastfeeding terms, "Why am I nursing my baby? Why do I want to breastfeed?"

Everyone's basic answer is because it is better than formula. Let's just unpack this. Breastmilk is species specific milk. If you worked in the San Diego Zoo and you were out of tiger milk, no one would suggest rhino milk. Rhinos and tigers have very different growth patterns and needs. You would not give a koala elephant milk. Yet no one seems to have a problem giving people cow milk. People are not cows! A baby calf needs to gain, two pounds A DAY, that is 620 pounds in its first year of life and be very sedated after it eats so as not to wander off and fall in a ditch somewhere. Baby humans need to grow their brains, and they need immune protection. First, let's talk about the brain. You are starting with a newborn who looks at you with focused eyes that at birth can see the distance from your breast to your face. What's happening across the room doesn't matter. It's all about you. Focus on this time since it is fleeting. When you have a sixteen year old, it will so not be about you, and focusing on Mom's face, unless she is holding food, is just not all that. In one short year these little people go from just seeing you to walking around with a cracker in one hand and a toy in the other saying a few words. That's a lot of brain development! If you want to know all the nitty gritty on how breastfed babies brains are fed with breastmilk check out the references in the back under How Breastmilk is Brainfood. On to immune support. No matter how many times I say this it always gives me goosebumps. When you pump the milk of women who have premature babies, they have specific ingredients in their milk to develop lung function that a Mom who gives birth to a full term infant never has in her milk. Your body knows your baby needs a little help in the breathing department and it provides! Everything you have ever been vaccinated against, every disease you have ever had all cause antibodies in your milk. Your baby gets them when he is nursing. And as he grows and nurses for less time, the immunity gets more concentrated in your milk. So your newborn nursing frequently is getting the same amount of immune protection as your one year old who nurses much less often and is eating food. Tell me you have goosebumps now.

I'm about to launch into the Benefits of Breastfeeding A-Z. Before you start flipping pages to get to the more juicy bits, hang on. When you feel like calling it quits at 3am, these benefits just might encourage you to keep going. They will help you remember that this is not just a fish or chicken choice between breastfeeding and formula. Breastmilk is species specific, in tune to the age of your baby and filled with LIVE white blood cells made by your body. We call it milk because that sounds nicer than let's feed our babies white blood cells, but you do not make a dairy product! You're human, and you make white blood cells. Compare this to something in a can. Now before you think I'm a formula hater, let's just clear something up. I am on the same page as the World Health Organization for infant feeding and its order of recommended infant nutrition: 1. Milk from the baby's own Mother. 2. Milk from another Mother. 3. Milk from a Milk Bank. 4. Formula. Formula, or as some people call it: artificial baby milk, is the fourth choice if nothing else is available. Any supplementation is just a tool to get nursing back on track - not the solution to the problem. Tires make the car go. But you can still turn the engine on without tires or even with a flat tire. I had to throw an analogy in there for the men reading this. Just saying, many interventions are simply tools to make breastfeeding work. So here we go with the A to Z benefits. If you have a group of women grab some chocolate, have everyone read one, or four; it is A to Z after all!

Amenorrhea, or a delay in the return of a Mother's menstrual cycle (once the approximately six weeks of lochia or postpartum bleeding and discharge has stopped), can last six months or longer in a

Mother who is exclusively breastfeeding her child. It is common for fertility to return between nine and eighteen months postpartum. Ovulation in non-lactating Mothers may occur as early as three weeks postpartum. The Lactational Amenorrhea Method (LAM) is ninety-eight to ninety-nine percent effective in avoiding another pregnancy when three conditions are met: your baby is younger than six months old, your periods haven't resumed, and your baby is breastfeeding exclusively and on cue day and night without regularly receiving any other food or drink, including water.

This is one of my favorite benefits of breastfeeding: no period. Cheer! You have enough going on without dealing with Aunt Rose. Does anyone call their period that anymore? One of the other factors besides the three above is not going more than a single four-hour stretch in twenty-four hours without nursing. One is fine. More than one every day for a week or two can signal your body to ovulate. As a public service announcement, I would like to state that you ovulate BEFORE you menstruate. So it is possible to not have a period and get pregnant. Just so we are clear it is possible to get pregnant, though the odds are not likely, if your baby is between six weeks and six months. So if you absolutely without a doubt DO NOT want to get pregnant, I suggest a NON hormonal form of birth control. Many women say the mini pill is fine for breastfeeding, but there are no long term studies that follow babies who were nursed while their Moms were taking birth control and then followed them on their own journey of fertility. For some women, even the mini pill affects their milk supply, and I have no idea if that's going to be you or not so I say non hormonal birth control is the safest choice for the first year. It is possible to not have your period for twenty-four months when the above rules are followed and you are nursing on demand.

Bonding through breastfeeding initially happens thanks to the release of prolactin and oxytocin, hormones responsible for the warm and motherly feeling that helps to bond a Mother to her newborn child. Often the loving bond is immediate, but sometimes this sense of love takes time to grow.

This is a no brainer. Bonding is increased with breastfeeding. Imagine you and your husband were face to face and hip to hip every two hours during the day and night for six weeks. You would know, that face means more coffee, that face means hurry up, that face means I need some space. But seriously, when you spend time, close time, with someone you get to know them. You have waited to meet this person for nine months! And in some cases you have been trying to get pregnant with this person for much longer than that, so enjoy spending some time with him. Even with lots of visitors and baby being passed around you are the one who can nurse your baby, and for Moms who plan to return to work this is a very special connection at the end of the day!

Colostrum is the perfect first food. It's the milk you produce in small amounts in the first couple of days after your baby is born. It has concentrated immunological properties that are your baby's first protection against germs as well as protection and repair for the delicate and vulnerable newborn intestine. Colostrum also acts as a laxative to help baby pass the first stool, meconium, which has a tar-like consistency and is composed of substances that the baby ingested in the womb.

Colostrum is THICK, think the thickest milkshake you can imagine. It is like primer to paint your baby's intestines to keep any germs out. If your baby is newborn and is not nursing well, ask for a spoon. It comes sterile wrapped in plastic on every food tray. You can hand express (more on that later) some into a spoon. A feeding for a newborn is just a teaspoon and the more colostrum you remove in the first twenty-four hours the sooner and better your milk comes in. I know it seems like reverse logic, but the emptier your breasts are the faster you're making milk. The fuller your breasts are the slower you will make milk. Otherwise, you would just get fuller and fuller until you were Pamela Anderson meets Dolly Parton, and then you would pop. No one wants to pop, unless it's a well placed color accessory to your outfit.

Meconium is your baby's first poo; it's tar-like and super sticky. It should only last a day or four days at the most, after the first few days you will have some transitional stool with traces of meconium in them. They could be brown or green, and then they change to a mustard yellow color. Many people seem to give colostrum a bad rap these days. They say "well my milk isn't in, and all I have is colostrum." Remember this is the first thing your baby has ever eaten besides amniotic fluid. It's the warm up for the milk. It's in the perfect amount, and there is nothing less than about it. I think when talking about colostrum it's all about the punctuation. Really! You could say, "Let's eat Grandma!" or "Lets eat, Grandma!" So instead of I have colostrum, It's I HAVE colostrum!!!! Cue the fireworks and air horn!

Decreased risk of breast cancer—possibly from the lower estrogen level of lactation—has been found in various studies. The longer a Mother breastfeeds, the less susceptible she is to breast, uterine, and cervical cancer.

Yes people, decreased cancer risk! Also, if you have a girl baby and nurse at least a year you also decrease her risk for breast cancer. Nothing else does that!

Easy baby care. Breastfeeding is always available and requires no additional equipment. Your baby controls the amount of milk intake at a feeding, and since breastfeeding is based on supply and demand, you produce the amount of milk your baby needs to get through growth spurts and any other time. No need to be somewhere to be able to make bottles. You are ready when the baby needs you.

Breast milk is always the right temp; It is always sterile and never runs out. I have nursed on the tarmac while our flight had to have the cockpit window replaced, and it took three hours. When we landed and got up the people behind us said, "We didn't even know you had a baby there did you drug him?" I said, "No, I just nursed him," thinking they have no idea what milk drunk is. I have also nursed on the side of a ski slope, on countless theme park rides, on trains, buses…It starts to sound like a children's book: I nursed in a box with a fox, on a plane in the rain! If you are worried about nursing in public, try first in a changing room. It has a bench, a big mirror and you can see what other people see from the front view, which is mainly your baby's head. This is where a baby sling can come in super handy. I think besides diapers, a baby sling or carrier is essential to having easy baby care. It lets your baby be close to you and thus the right temp. It keeps your baby in your personal space so strangers are less likely to touch him, and it's a whole lot lighter than that heavy car seat. Which I would like to point out is called CAR SEAT, not baby carrier! Those things weigh a ton and really do a number on your abs that are trying to recover from being so far out from their normal position. Wear your baby. Your baby, your abs, and I will thank you. And you encourage other people to nurse in public and wear their babies too. Attitude is everything! If you are feeding your baby in public, don't hide yourself! You are not doing anything that women have not done for thousands of years. Hold your head high and smile. Who knows? That grandma giving you the eye may be going to go home and tell her daughter in law, "I saw the most amazing thing in Target today!" That is how nursing in public changes to being the norm. Be the change ladies; it starts with you!

Few allergies come from breast milk. Human milk is non-allergenic. There is a possibility of something the Mother consumes passing to her breastfeeding child, so if a family has a history of allergies with specific foods, the Mother may choose to introduce those foods into her diet slowly. By far the safest, healthiest food for your baby is your milk.

Before you start freaking out thinking that you need to eat a special diet while you are breastfeeding, let me reassure you, you don't. When you think of women all over the world nursing babies you realize Mothers in Mexico having chilis and salsa with their meals do not have a country of fussy babies! In the same way Mothers in China having cabbage and broccoli do not have a country of gassy babies. In Italy, having garlic on food does not produce colicky bambinos! It is the exact opposite. Your milk takes on the subtle flavors of what you eat. So Moms in India who are eating curry have milk with a subtle curry flavor. When their babies start solids with curry, it seems familiar to them. You can take out curry and replace it with any favorite food: thai chili paste, mango chutney, or fish and chips with malt vinegar! So eat up! Now, if you have a family history of allergies, for example, if your husband eats shellfish and swells up like a puffer fish, then you might want to avoid shellfish until your baby is six months months old. Things that pass into breast milk are things with a big protein molecule. In no particular order they are: nuts, soy, eggs, dairy, and shellfish. Usually eaten in moderation these are not a problem. But when you have an overload, it can make your baby fussy or or give him an eczema type rash, including diaper rash.

When in doubt you can do this simple test. Consider the offending food. Dairy seems to be the most common on the list, so start with that if you're not sure. For one week completely eliminate dairy. Then after the week have a dairy fest. Go all out with cereal with milk, grilled cheese for lunch and ice cream or a milkshake as a snack. If after or during your dairy fest your baby then has a total fussy freak out, the rash comes back, or symptoms begin to increase again, then it probably is dairy. To be absolutely super sure, you can eliminate the dairy for two weeks and see if all the symptoms go away. If on the other hand, after your dairy fest, your baby is just as fussy as the week of no dairy, it's probably not dairy. You can try something else on the list. However, I have known women to get down to eating nothing but white bread and potatoes because they think that everything they are eating is making their baby fussy when in reality they just have a fussy baby. If it is not one of the above mentioned allergy items and you don't have a family history, it's probably not a food allergy.

If it did turn out to be a food allergy then good news, after your baby is six months old their gut junctures start to close up. Before six months they are like the holes in a strainer; after they are more like bricks in a wall. Cue the Pink Floyd song, "We don't need no, allergic babies." Ok, maybe you're not a Pink Floyd fan. Anyway, after six months try to add in the offending food a little at a time to your diet and see. If you notice a reaction, wait until one year to try again. Also, be careful giving the offending food to your baby directly once they are ready for solids. If they are having a reaction through breast milk, the reaction will likely be even stronger when they have the food directly. To sum up: eat whatever you want while breastfeeding. If you think something you're eating is bothering your baby, take it out of your diet for a week, then eat a ton of it and watch what happens. The good news is your breast milk changes taste based on what you are eating, so it is an eating adventure for your baby everyday. This makes breastfed babies start to solids semi familiar and not too new. Formula is vanilla flavor at best so only having the same bottle of vanilla makes that first bite of sweet potatoes seem shocking.

Good for the whole family. Breastfeeding not only helps raise healthier babies, it also models that babies are important and need to be nursed and held close a lot. I also think it helps to continue growing the rates of breastfeeding. If your children see breastfeeding as natural, they will use the same method to feed their babies. Also, hormones that are released while breastfeeding - like oxytocin - help Mothers recover faster, sleep better, and overall be happier. Happy Mothers equal happy families.

Breastfed babies are healthier for a huge number of reasons. One of the most fascinating reasons is, when you breathe in the germs around you, you then make antibodies to those germs and the antibodies appear in your milk. Amazing! So if you're in Target and someone coughs on you and your baby, never fear, within minutes you will produce antibodies in your milk for that cough. Now, if Dad took your baby to Home Depot so you could nap, and someone coughs on them, this doesn't work. In a recent study of Moms who took their babies to daycare, both groups of babies were getting pumped milk at daycare. The Moms who nursed on pick up and drop off in the daycare room had babies that were less sick than those getting pumped milk only. Antibodies people, it's amazing!

Human milk is specially designed for human babies. Many families never drink cow's or goat's milk. Other milks aren't necessary for humans, but if you plan to introduce anything other than breastmilk it is a good idea to wait until your baby is one year old in order to reduce the risk of allergies.

Your baby does not need anything but human milk for the first six months. No water, no fluoride, no iron, no Vitamin D. While breast milk is low in iron compared to formula, the iron it does have is easily absorbed. Breast milk also changes depending on your baby's age to be the perfect milk for the age of your baby.

IgAs are the specific molecules that are in breastmilk that keep the gut flora with more good guys than bad guys. Secretory IgA molecules further keep an infant from harm in that, unlike most other antibodies, they ward off disease without causing inflammation - a process in which various chemicals destroy microbes but potentially hurt healthy tissue.

If you haven't picked up on this yet, breastmilk is alive! They look at pumped milk and test the bacteria levels when it is freshly pumped, then check it again six hours later, and it's lower in bacteria than when it's first pumped! It actually eats its own bacteria. So your milk can stay at room temperature from six to eight hours without going bad. You can also use a bottle of milk again if your baby did not finish it for this same reason. This is why I do not suggest mixing breastmilk and formula in the same bottle, because you have to throw it out if it's more than just breast milk. Also, since breast milk has antibodies it works to clean up a goopy eye in an infant. Simply express a drop into a spoon and use a clean eye dropper to place a drop in the corner of your infants eye. I usually suggest this at each diaper change. Your baby's sticky goopy eye should clear up in a day.

Jaw development is broader in your breastfed child compared to the jaw that results from bottle-feeding and pacifiers. While breastfeeding, the baby's jaw muscles are exercised and massaged in a way that causes the bones in your baby's face and jaw to develop more fully. Narrow jaw development may restrict nose breathing, cause snoring, or require orthodontia later on.

For me, nothing is as handsome as a strong jawline. I am looking at you Brad Pitt. But seriously, in a case study of two, my own children, here is how it went down. I do not have perfect teeth; my husband does not have perfect teeth. There was not a braces fund left for me as I am last on the birth order of four. So you cannot say that my children inherited perfect teeth. Yet they both have movie star teeth! My oldest even has room for his wisdom teeth to come in. The only way I can explain this is breastfeeding. Neither one of my children used a pacifier or had bottles. So their palate and jaw developed without any hard plastic molding them. Dr. Brian Palmer DDS looked at a bunch of caveman skulls and talks about how jaw development changed with bottle feeding. All of the caveman skulls had their teeth aligned and with plenty of room. Check out his work, it's fascinating! If not for health reasons, let's just look at the money savings alone. Google cost of braces…I'll wait. Yeah, and what came up was probably the coupon bargain price as your first hit. You can save this by nursing your baby. With the savings you can buy yourself a really nice purse, and come out ahead. Way ahead. Really. I did.

Kids get lots of attention when the new baby is breastfed. When your baby is hungry, you can continue doing whatever you were doing with the older kids and nurse rather than preparing a bottle. It also means only the Mother feeds the baby, so when Dad is home, he can give more attention to older kids instead of sharing feeding duties.

Multitasking is a nursing Mom's best strategy. This is true if you have more than one child. You have one free hand to read a book, or cuddle another little one. If this is your first baby you can use that other hand to hold your own book, Kindle, burrito, granola bar, remote…you get the idea. Eating one handed snacks is important in the early weeks. Wraps are great as well as a good old fashioned sandwiches. Hard boiled eggs, already peeled, cut up veggies, and fruits are also great one hand wonders.

Laundry is a breeze. The sun can remove most breastfed stool stains left behind on clean laundry. Unless it is treated with a really good stain remover, formula spit up can stain clothing brown.

With a new baby there is a lot of laundry but breast milk spit up, leaked milk on clothes, and breast milk poo are all washable. No special stain removers needed. To keep laundry simple just let the socks and undies stay in the basket and get them from there, no need to fold. Having anyone who is there to help you take over the laundry is always a welcome task for both of you! They feel useful and you don't have to worry about it. Spending the first weeks in your pjs or some easy loungewear also keeps the laundry to a minimum and keeps you in a rest mode, and says to visitors, you are in recovery mode not hostess mode.

Mental development is normal in breastfed babies but is linked to lower IQ scores in formula-fed babies. Breastfeeding doesn't automatically add IQ points, but research indicates the longer a child breastfeeds the higher his intelligence.

Breastfeeding grows brains. If you think of what a human baby needs to know in the first year it's a TON of brain growth. Sitting up, crawling, walking all give a different visual perspective on the world and babies will usually want to nurse more during these times. Nursing is the safe place. All the rest of this is new and can be scary. That's why I like to call it nursing and not breastfeeding. When your baby is at the breast they are feeling your heartbeat pulse through your nipple. They are feeling the rise and fall of your chest, and they are smelling the smell of your colostrum and milk which is the same smell as your amniotic fluid. One group of researchers put expressed milk on nursing pads of the baby's own Mother on one pad and another Mom's milk on another pad and put them on either side of a baby. The baby turned toward the pad with his Mom's milk on it. You are doing so much more than providing a transfer of nutrition. You are creating a safe space, a place where when the doorbell is ringing and the dog is barking there is not a need to freak out because this smell, this heartbeat, this breathing pattern is known and familiar, and is safe. This security is brain building in a way that says to your baby someone is present, and cares for me, and I can trust her.

Natural is the key word. Breast milk requires no manufacturing equipment, preparation, or artificial methods. "Human milk has many hundreds of known and unknown ingredients, including interferon and white blood cells, antibacterial and antiviral agents, intestinal soothers, growth hormones, and everything else a baby is known to need."

Your body makes milk effortlessly. It has grown your baby for nine months; and it's not just going to ditch you on the breastfeeding thing. Nursing frequently in the early days is the single most important thing you can do to make this natural process work. What gets in the way of the natural is intervention. Separating Mom and baby at birth, not being an active and alert participant in childbirth, and letting baby sleep for longer than three hours all throw a stick in the wheel of what is natural. A speaker at an online conference in Australia said they are changing the suggested nursing sessions in a twenty-four hour period from eight to ten times as we have here in the U.S to thirteen to sixteen in twenty-four hours! I think this is because if you say to a new Mom nurse ten to twelve they might get eight to ten.   If you say thirteen to sixteen then you will get ten to twelve. Babies need to nurse every two hours during the day and every three hours at night. This timing is start time to start time, and YES, there will be feeds that run together. I call daytime from 5 am to 11 pm and night time from 11 pm to 5 am. We will talk about cluster feeds and growth spurts later along with hunger cues. For now, let's just focus on infant gut capacity. Your baby has a stomach the size of a marble at birth, that's why a teaspoon of colostrum is enough at that age. Then it goes to the size of a ping pong ball from two weeks to about six months. Look at your baby's fist; that's about the size of their stomach. So your baby eats, then they poo, then they are ready to eat again. This is also a survival tool. Breast milk is super easy for your baby to digest, and since he needs to eat often, you are also checking in with him to see if he is too hot or too cold, if he is breathing normally, if he needs to spit up or cough. When he is on his side not his back nursing it makes him less likely to choke. The natural position for nursing is your baby on his side.This is also a great position for airway clearing.

Oxytocin and prolactin are nature's way of encouraging a Mother's body to take care of her baby and to transition from birth by stimulating uterine contractions. With each feeding, the hormones are released for milk let down and to foster feelings of love and nurturing. Without these hormones, Mothers tend to talk to their babies less, interact less, and touch less.

The hormones of breastfeeding often called the mothering hormones tell you what to do as a Mom. They sharpen your Mom instincts to understand cries and get to know your baby. They also relax you to sleep and nurse with your baby. If Betty Sue cave woman got a burst of adrenaline when she nursed she would have cut the nursing session short and gone out and swept the cave, hunted and skinned dinner and had a cave party. But instead she just took a nap with her baby. I can relate. If nursing and napping were an Olympic sport I would have gotten a gold medal. Really. It is how I survived the newborn period.

Protection against your baby becoming obese, and getting breast cancer as well as other types of cancer.

Research shows that nursing your baby lowers his risk for obesity, and when your child grows up, he is not an overweight adult. His risk is lower for the other cancers he could have if he were obese such as pancreatic, endometrial, esophageal, rectal and kidney cancers. There is a ton of research about this on the MD Anderson web site. You can also reduce the Mom's risk of breast cancer and ovarian cancer. The more you nurse the more your risk decreases. In one study, women who nursed multiple children for over thirty-one months reduced their risk of ovarian cancer by ninety-one percent compared to women who breastfed for ten months or under. Before you freak out about thirty-one months think about if you had three children and nursed them all for just a year. Done. Also nursing a one year old who eats a half of a half of a sandwich is different than just nursing a newborn who is only getting your milk.

You can find more about this in the websites/links and research section in the back of the book.

Quick weight loss from the hips and thighs can occur for Mothers when they breastfeed— something women are less able to do at other times.

Most women lose the most weight when their baby is six to twelve months old. You put on weight during pregnancy specifically for nursing. So if you were in the cave and ran out of mammoth jerky you would still make milk for your baby. When you see pictures of third world countries with Moms who are severely malnourished their breastfed babies look great! It's the weaned toddlers who have the distended belly and shallow faces. After six months your body knows your baby is starting to eat solids and then you start to shed that weight. You can lose up to a pound a week without dieting and exercise, just nursing! That's my kinda weight loss! I gained seventy pounds with my first child, and with all the bouncing and walking that was needed to keep him from screaming at the top of his lungs, in an earth shattering way, I lost it all in the first year. Yep. I was back to my pre baby self. I can say he sucked it right out of me. Insert laughing emoji here.

Rest comes to breastfeeding mothers who breastfeed exclusively because they are in a hormonal state that facilitates sleep and allows them to respond to their baby's needs without fully waking up.

Resting and nursing makes baby care go smoother. There is a lot more to this to come but you actually get into the same sleep cycle as your baby when you are in the same airspace. James McKenna has amazing Mom and baby sleep lab and has lots of research online about how these sleep cycles work. You can find more about this in the websites/links and research section in the back of the book.

Saves money. Breastfeeding is free and is a renewable resource. Not every breastfeeding mother requires supplies, but if she does these products are usually one-time purchases.

You can really get it down to the basics when you have diapers, wipes and breasts. You don't need to pump milk to leave your baby, you just use timing. Aim to nurse your baby fully, so they are super full when you leave them to go to Target. Believe it or not there are Moms who go back to work and they don't pump at all. Their caregiver brings the baby to them to nurse or they have an on site day care where they can pop in nurse and get back to work. The baby will always be faster and more efficient at taking out milk, than any pump will. Believe me if there was a pump company that could do that then their ads would be all over the place...Better than your baby, It's the Pumpzilla!

Traveling is easy since breastfeeding can mean instant comfort in any location.

If you go on vacation somewhere and your baby is not into trying the local cuisine then you can be comforted he will still be able to have your milk. If you have travelers diarrhea or even food poisoning your milk remains safe and sound.

Understanding your baby's needs becomes instinctive.

With each day you get to know your baby better, and as they get head control around six weeks, nursing gets much easier and you understand that nursing is more than food, it's an all purpose comfort tool.

Vitamins and minerals and other nutritional elements that your baby's body needs, including many that haven't been discovered or named yet, are contained in human milk and can subtly change through a nursing session, day, or year to match your baby's needs

With every year that goes by more and more research is going into what is in breast milk. And it continues to astound researchers. I just went to a conference where the speaker mentioned the discovery of over two-hundred fatty acids alone in breastmilk. You don't need to worry that you are eating perfectly. I suggest eating foods as close to their natural state as possible. Try for some omega 3 rich foods like tuna fish or sushi or smoked salmon on a bagel. Also having a green smoothie is a great way to get your dose of fruits and veggies. I recently subscribed to a smoothie delivery service called Daily Harvest. They deliver frozen cups of goodness to your door. All you do is dump the contents in a blender, add your liquid and pour them back into the cup they came in. Lid with straw hole included! These would be great for new Moms, or you can have anyone who is helping you prep bags of frozen smoothie goodness into your freezer. There are also many meal delivery services and of course grocery delivery. If only that was around when my babies were babies! Now is the time for all that delivery. Before you know it your baby will be in school, and you will have all the time in the world to go to the grocery and squeeze the peaches yourself to pick the perfect ripeness.

For now, leave that to someone else and nurse and nap.

Working goes smoothly when the nursing relationship is maintained. If you pump in the morning before work, you can bring that milk to the caregiver for the first morning feeding. If possible, your baby should still feed on demand and not on a schedule. If your baby becomes hungry towards the end of the work day, caregivers can give a small feeding of your expressed milk, knowing that you can nurse and reconnect with your baby when you arrive for pick up.

Working and nursing is possible. You don't need a Y2K storage facility of milk if you're planning on working. The milk you pump the day before can be used the next day. There is a great book on Working and Nursing called. "Nursing Mother, Working Mother " by Gale Pryor. This book is not new, but I love it and continue to suggest it because it talks about many different ways to combine working and nursing. While working and breastfeeding is possible, the key is gradually getting back to work. If you can go back to work slowly, either by a few hours a day, or a few days a week your body and baby will adjust better. Many women find that having their caregiver bring the baby to them to nurse at lunch makes one less pumping session and the baby gets some much needed Mom time. I also suggest the video Paced Bottle Feeding on Youtube. You can find more about this in the websites/links and research section in the back of the book. It really explains how to bottle feed a breastfed baby. Bottles just drip into your baby's mouth, and they have to swallow rapidly without a break to protect their airway. The only thing I can compare it to is beer bonging. The fluid is coming, and you have to keep swallowing! Paced bottle feeding prevents over feeding and allows your baby to just take what they want. They may be nursing because they are just thirsty, or a little hungry or super hungry! A sample schedule might look like this: Set your alarm for thirty minutes before you need to get up for work, nurse in bed. Then get up and shower and get dressed, nurse again. Eat breakfast, pack up your pump and your baby's bag and nurse right before you leave for the day care. Nurse at the daycare when you arrive, to breathe in any germs and make antibodies to them. So basically you leave your baby stuffed like a tick. If you pressed on them fluid would come seeping out. Now they can go their four hour stretch. So if you dropped them off at 9 am then they would be good till about lunch. Nurse them at lunch if you can go to them or they come to you. If not pump at lunch. Now this gets you to 3 pm. Pump a bottle and they will get a bottle of milk at daycare. This is your milk for the next day. Then you see them as soon as you get to the daycare at 5-ish and they are ready to nurse. This is just a sample schedule to give you an idea. But take it slow if at all possible. Wearing your baby in carrier or sling then giving that to your caregiver lets them carry your baby around in something that smells like you. This can help them feel like you are still near and give your caregiver another way to comfort them besides food.

Xactly what baby needs. Even if your child isn't hungry, breastfeeding almost always ends up being the solution for a fussy baby or toddler. Nursing is soothing.

What are some of the reasons you go out to eat? You want that kind of food? You have a coupon? You don't want to cook? You don't want to clean? We could list many more reasons why people go out to eat. What if you said you only go out to eat for a transfer of nutrition? Then we could just sit in the parking lot of the most expensive restaurant in town with IV nutrition in our arms and think we were having the time of our lives! Babies are the same. They want to nurse for all kinds of reasons. And many of those reasons are fixed by nursing. For example, they are too hot, nursing fixes that, too cold, nursing fixes that, over stimulated or under stimulated, nursing fixes that, they need to poo or they just pooped and it freaked them out, nursing fixes that. So when you think, they can't want to nurse. They are not hungry. Just think of all the other reasons to nurse like the reasons you want to go out to eat. Imagine your husband saying we can't go out to eat. We have food here.

You get to take care of your baby. Nursing is a normal follow-up to birth for the Mother as her body has been preparing to feed her baby. There are many ways Dads can help besides feeding the baby.

The book "The Womanly Art of Breastfeeding" where all of the above benefits come from, has a great section on Partners. Dads and other support people can do a lot to help the nursing Mother besides feed the baby. If you are bringing the nursing Mom food then you are feeding the baby. Then there are diapers, lots of diapers. Changes of clothes, burping, soothing. Did I mention diapers? Also, skin to skin is great! Try wearing a button up shirt and putting the baby inside with head nestled under your chin. I like to put the Not the Nursing Person in charge of bath time. This is their time to do it, their way, and to figure it out alone. One Mom did this, and it was so quiet in the bathroom she peeked in to see her husband using baby wipes to give the baby a bath. Hey, that works! It does not matter how they get clean, if there is peace or screaming, let them figure it out and find their way. They will get it, and this will be their special time. It may be bumpy at first giving a person with no head control a bath but soon that person will be laughing and splashing them back. Bath time is a great bonding time.

Zero waste. With direct breastfeeding there is no need for bottles, pacifiers, cans of anything or added water. So there is less waste going into the trash or using energy to be recycled.

Breast milk is the ultimate in living off the grid. You don't need electricity to make it, and there is no cost. You actually save enough money in one year of breastfeeding to buy a super fancy washer and dryer. Healthier babies mean less doctor's visits and less sick days for working Moms. Breast milk also is unlimited in supply and comes in attractive packaging; it never is recalled, never gets contaminated, and never expires. Power outage, no problem! You've got this!

Chapter Two:
Normal vs Needs Attention

Now that we have some basic knowledge under our belt from hearing about the benefits of nursing, let's use that to see if the following situations are Normal or they Need Attention. Again, if you want to do this in a game format then just read each situation and see if you can answer normal or needs attention. You can even have prizes! Ready? Lets go!

My baby won't take a bottle: Normal or Needs Attention?

Normal! There are many ways to feed a baby. If the baby is a newborn try a spoon, or a periodontal syringe. A flexible cup or a shot glass size cup can be used with any age baby. You simply hold baby upright and put the milk to their lips by tilting the cup, they will lap at the milk. There are many videos of this on Youtube. Just search cup feeding newborn. You can also use a periodontal syringe with your finger, pad side up. Make sure baby has his lips flanged out like fish lips and the seal is tight on your finger. If you hear slurping sounds lift the pad of your finger and press gently on the baby's pallet. To get him to suck make a come here motion with your finger. Then slip in the syringe about 2 cm, about the thickness of two credit cards, into his mouth. If you go too far with the syringe then you will pull their lip and it will break the suction. So get the syringe in enough to not spill out of his mouth but not so far in that you're breaking the seal. Then start pushing the plunger of the syringe. You should feel the milk pool around your finger like you are filling a tiny teacup. When you feel the milk pooling, stop plunging, let baby swallow. Go slow to avoid spilling. One and a half ounces to two ounces should take about fifteen to twenty minutes. Watch the baby for signs of stress, clenched fists, furrowed brow, turning away are all stress signs. This technique can also be used to feed a baby who is not latching well, is sleepy at the breast, or who needs some extra milk to gain weight. Sometimes, giving the baby one-fourth of an ounce before the feed can organize them if they are too fussy to latch on. Think of it as a appetizer course before the main entrée.

My baby spits up: Normal or Needs Attention?

Babies spit up. That is normal. If you have a happy spitter, the one who spits up and smiles as milk comes out of their mouth you have nothing to worry about. As your baby gets used to nursing and understands how much sucking equals how much milk then they will stop before they are too full. Also, when babies are born their esophageal tube does not fully seal into their stomach. Think of it as a cup with the lid open a little. So if you have a super full baby and you lay him down right away, his cup will overflow. Milk isn't that heavy, and there is such a short distance in babies from their stomach compared to an older child or adult. Keeping your baby upright after meals for fifteen minutes, or even just not moving them around right after they eat can really help. The big issue with spit up is reflux. Reflux in its worst form is a baby who is spitting up more than they are gaining. These babies look anything but happy. I have only seen one of these in fifteen years and it was not a case where you had to wonder if something was going wrong. This baby spit up cups of milk, and spent over half of their day being miserable. So to sum up if you have a happy spitter rejoice; if your baby seems miserable, first try taking out all dairy from your diet, in many cases this will solve the problem. Second, try for shorter more frequent feeds. Just like when you were nine months pregnant you could not eat a ton of food at each meal and go a long time between meals. Shorter more frequent feeds may help your baby keep what he takes in down better. Please keep reading to understand how to check your baby for tongue tie, when your baby is popping on and off the breast and not making a complete seal because of their oral anatomy they will take in air, this can look like reflux, but it is actually tongue tie or a disorganized suck.

My breasts are uncomfortably huge - they feel heavy, hard, and hot like they might pop: Normal or Needs Attention?

Needs attention! This is engorgement and can be normal if it lasts an hour to twenty-four hours. Many women find they are engorged for days or even weeks and this is NOT NORMAL! Here is what to do! First, nurse your baby. If your nipple is too tight and flat due to the swelling try and hand express some milk. There are a ton of videos on hand expression. I like the ones from Stanford the best, but just watch till you find one that works. I could list the instructions here but it's more of a visual thing, so you might need to watch someone do it. You can also use a pump for one to three minutes to take the pressure off. When your milk comes in, It. COMES. IN. It starts when the placenta detaches from the uterus and your body says this baby is out. We need to start making milk to feed it. The problem is your body does not know if you had one baby, or three babies, so you make milk for about two babies in the beginning. Nursing frequently will help regulate your supply. Your baby does a much better job of this than a pump does, as when the breast is comfortable, and the baby leaves some milk in there, then your body says Ok, let's not make that much the next time. Over the next six weeks your baby will drive the supply, and your body will make the perfect amount of milk for your baby right as your baby needs it. This is why milk removal is so important in the first twenty-four hours. The more colostrum you remove; the more it sends the signal to your breasts to make milk. So your first line of defense against engorgement is nursing. If you are still full after that you can try a cold compress, I like a bag of frozen peas to take the hotness down. You can also try taking an over the counter anti inflammatory like Advil. If after forty-eight to seventy-two hours of frequent nursing, nursing every thirty minutes to one hour, you are still having engorgement then you can try some cabbage. There is an enzyme in green cabbage that passes through your skin and decreases your milk supply. In one study, they tried to give women cabbage pills and nothing happened. So here is how you do it. Take a head of green cabbage and peel the leaves off and wrap your breast in it like a mummy costume. Wrapping all over and covering the whole breast top, sides, nipple and bottom. You are going to need to put up your bra flaps to hold all the leaves on. So flaps up and let it sit for a while till it wilts. After about two hours, when it is done it should be like cooked cabbage. If you can put your finger nail in it and it crunches then its not done. Cabbage can be powerful so you only want to do it once, maybe twice a day to see how it's going to affect you. Set a timer, don't fall asleep with it in. Ask me how I know this.

My baby is two weeks old. Today he has had one wet diaper and he has not had a soiled diaper in three days: Normal or Needs Attention?

This needs attention. Breastfed babies should have six to ten wet diapers and at least two to four soiled diaper in twenty-four hours after day six. Six wet and two soiled are on the low side. Many babies stool at every feeding. To count as a soiled diaper, after your milk comes in, the poo needs to be at least two quarters worth. If you put two quarters in the diaper the poo should cover that. Less than is just gas with a bonus. In the early days of life number of diapers go with days of life. So on day 1, its one wet diaper and one soiled diaper.   On day 2, it is two wet and one soiled. day 3, it is three wet and one soiled. Day 4, four wet and one soiled. Day 5, five wet and one soiled. By day 5 your milk should have really come in, and this is where it changes. After day 6, you should have six to ten wet and two to four soiled in twenty-four hours. There are a few cases where Mom's milk comes in on day 7 or even day 10, but those are rare cases. The first thing to look at is how much is your baby nursing? If they are nursing ten to twelve times in twenty-four hours then that is a good amount. The next thing to do is see an International Board Certified Lactation Consultant. An IBCLC has Health Science education, Lactation Specific clinical experience, and Lactation specific education. Depending on what pathway they certified with, they had to have 300 to 1000 of supervised lactation hours. They are also required to have 75 Continuing Education requirements every five years and sit the board certified exam every ten years. This is a four hour proctored exam done by an independent test organization with slides and questions. All IBCLC's have had college level health science courses.

In contrast a certified lactation consultant or CLC must only take 20-120 hours of classroom training, and pass a written exam offered by the training organization. They only have to have a high school diploma, and they do not have to have ANY hands on hours working with Moms and babies. It is important to know the difference in these because you could pay the same amount of money to see a CLC as an IBCLC and have a very different outcome. Also, the CLC is not required to send a note to your pediatrician or midwife detailing your visit and care plan, and the IBCLC is required to do this.

If you are in the low diaper count situation described above, the IBCLC will weigh your baby, help you get into a good position to nurse your baby, and then weigh your baby again. The scale I use to do this weighs to the one one hundredth of an ounce. This will give a snapshot of what your baby's intake is. The IBCLC will ask you if this is a usual feed or the best academy award feeding your baby ever had. This gives you an idea of how this compares to how your baby usually nurses. Normal intake for a two week old is 2.0 oz. This based on normal infant gut capacity. For a younger baby, the normal transfer is as follows: first 24 - 48 hours of life: one teaspoon equals a feed so it's hard to do a test weight on these tiny people. On day three to five normal transfer is about half an ounce per feed, then on day five to seven it's .5 oz to 1.5 oz, then from day seven to two weeks it jumps to 2.0 oz - 2.5 oz per feed. These are the minimal ranges, your baby might take take slightly more, or slightly less, and still have normal gain and normal diaper output. In studies where they do twenty-four hours of test weights and weigh, nurse, weigh the baby after each feed, you will see the numbers be all over the place. Sometimes your baby is super hungry so it might be 2.5 oz as the transfer. Other times your baby is just thirsty so it will be just .5 oz to 1.0 oz. When the diapers are normal and baby is growing in an upward trend there is no need to obsess on the transfer. If the diapers are low, the transfer can give you an idea of what is going on. If the transfer is in the normal range, nursing more often and avoiding pacifiers really fixes the weight gain issue. I like to start with something simple then go to more complicated if needed. If nursing more doesn't work, adding in some pumping and giving the baby some pumped milk with the syringe while at the breast can be the boost that you need to get the diapers back on track. Your pumping output does not equal the amount of milk you can make. Some women just don't get a let down with the pump because the pump is not your baby. It's like making love to the toaster. It isn't cute, does not smell like anything or look at you lovingly! The pump is just a tool to use when your baby needs some extra help. There is a great video in the back section under websites and links called hands on pumping. Check it out if you need to boost your supply or you have an early baby.

My baby cries every night in the evening from 5-7 pm: Normal or Needs Attention?

This can be normal. It even has a name! Cluster feeding- this is a four hour stretch of time where your baby wants to nurse. Usually it happens in the evening but it can happen in the morning or at other times during the day as well. Your baby is tanking themselves up to sleep for a four hour stretch of time. I know I talked about nursing every two hours during the day and every three hours at night, but if your baby is growing normally with a good wet and soiled diaper count, then you can go four hours one time in twenty-four hours. I suggest you SLEEP during this time and not try and dust, load the dishwasher, be on your phone or computer or get anything done. Sleep when the baby sleeps is a good motto to keep you from going to crazy town. When you are not sleeping everything looks like a crisis. This goes for Moms, Dads and toddlers. When your baby is in a cluster feed this is the perfect time to binge on Netflix, catch up on Ellen, listen to books on audible or did I mention SLEEP!

My baby is six months old and I still haven't started my period: Normal or Needs Attention?

This is NORMAL, and I mainly put it in to see if you remember the first benefit we talked about. No period! Go back and reread that section. If your baby is six months or under and has not started solids yet and is exclusively breastfeeding you have the most fertility protection. Once your baby starts taking anything by mouth, bottle, pacifier, food, you need to consider another form of birth control if you want to avoid getting pregnant. There are some women who despite following all the rules get their period back, if you are worried and really don't want to get pregnant then, use condoms! If you are a woman who gets their period back, I give you permission to buy a new pair of shoes and eat some chocolate as

a consolation. Really, it sucks! Get on
Zappos right now.

My baby gags and chokes every time my
milk lets down and he is really gassy:
Normal or Needs Attention?

This is called overactive let down. Some of
the symptoms are spraying milk during the
let down, and then your baby eats their
entire 2.0 oz in less than five minutes. That
causes gas and fussiness since your milk
comes in a big gush, think fire hose, after
your baby has had a few sucks. Some people
can describe this as a pins and needles
feeling or a release feeling, or like your foot
is falling asleep, except the sensation is in
your breast, not your foot. The most simple
way to deal with this is take your baby off
your breast, let the milk spray into a diaper
or cloth or catch it in a cup and put your
baby back on. You can let your baby suck
on your finger as you are doing the catching
so they don't scream bloody murder having

being taken out of the restaurant while only having had a few sucks of their dinner. Another option is to lean back and get the line from your hip to your shoulder at a 90 degree angle. Then the milk has to flow uphill. You can also latch your baby on in the biological nurturing position where they are straddling your leg. Do a search for biological nurturing and then click the video for the full details.

I feel like I am getting the flu. My breast is sore and red, and I have a fever. My body aches all over: Normal or Needs Attention?

This is Mastitis and is NOT NORMAL. Mastitis is a breast infection. There are two types of Mastitis. Bacterial and viral. Bacterial happens when you have a cracked or open spot on your nipple, and germs get into your breast through the broken skin causing an infection. It is important if you have an open place on your nipple to use ONE DOT, I'm talking the size of two capital letters on a page, like this (OO) amount of polysporin. It's also Polysporin with a P NOT Neosporin! Sold right next to the Neosporin at the drug or grocery store. I just am re-reading this and the (OO) amount guide I gave you looks like two breasts. I think I just invented an emoji! Ok, back to business. Bacterial Mastitis has a cut or open place, and you have a fever and chills and body aches. It really does feel like you have the flu, except your breast hurts and is red. You need to treat the bacterial one with antibiotics topically and orally from your OB. The viral type is when you have all of the above: fever, red breast, stripe of red on your breast or red spot and flu like symptoms with painful breast. If you catch this early and you see a major improvement in your symptoms in twenty-four hours you don't need antibiotics. Step one: get in bed with your baby and nurse! Not getting the milk out is the major cause of this type of Mastitis. It is like you and I went on a road trip for fourteen hours, and your husband was driving and did not want to stop, and we were drinking thirty-two ounces of water. After a certain point your bladder can only hold so much, so we would get bladder infections. Your breast can only involute so much milk before there is nowhere for the milk to go. So skipping a feed, wearing a too tight bra that causes the milk to not be able to leak out, can all be mastitis triggers. But the main causes of Mastitis are not getting the milk out and fatigue! So nurse often and NAP! There is no way you can get all the sleep you need in one night, so you must nap. Step two: drink one 8 oz glass of water an hour, to keep things flowing.

My baby is eight weeks old and he has not had a stool in three days; the last time he did have a soiled diaper it was soft and pasty not seedy like it used to be: Normal or Needs Attention?

This is normal, as your baby gets past six weeks the diapers start to slow down a little. The texture can still be in a wide range of normal from total liquid to paste and everything in between. However, a baby who is only getting breastmilk should never have a formed hard poo. If you can pop out the poo like a dog turd and fling it and when it lands it is still in the same shape then that's just not right. The biggest question I get is: Is my baby having diarrhea? When your breastfed baby has an intestinal virus the poo will smell rank. I can't really describe it, but it smells like sickness, think rancid meat. If you have to smell it over and over to decide, it's not that. People entering the room with the diaper on and locked and loaded would say, "What is that smell?!"

I don't know what people mean by let down, I don't feel anything and my breasts don't leak: Normal or Needs Attention?

This can be normal. Most women will notice breast changes during their pregnancy and when their milk comes in. However, after your milk supply equalizes, around six weeks you may feel your breast to be a lot like your pre-pregnant state. You body is just making milk when your baby needs it, exactly at the time your baby eats, and the perfect amount. Many Mothers notice a fuller feeling when they are outside in hot weather. We are in Texas, so I'm talking 100 degrees here. Hot where you live may mean 80 degrees. Your body knows that you are hot, so your baby must be hot also so it starts making thin milk to satisfy thirst. Amazing right?!

My baby has white patches in his mouth and a diaper rash that won't clear up. I'm getting a sharp stabbing pain even when I'm not even nursing him and I currently have a vaginal yeast infection: Normal or Needs Attention?

Needs attention! This is thrush! It is a yeast infection on your nipples. Many things can spark it such as: Having IV antibiotics during or after delivery- This kills off bacteria, bad as well as good, and the yeast can get out of hand without the good bacteria. If you do need IV antibiotics for delivery or due to group B strep, be sure to take a probiotic along with them. Another cause of thrush is sitting in wet nursing pads or bra, especially in hot weather. This is like a invitation for thrush. You have all of its favorite things, dark, wet, sticky, hot; it's the perfect environment for thrush! To get rid of thrush you need to treat Mom AND BABY AT THE SAME TIME. Sorry for the all caps, but this is something that I say over and over, and over and over again and STILL I have to keep saying it. If one of you has thrush and you are putting your nipple with thrush or the mouth with thrush together twelve times a day you are just going to keep passing it back and forth, and back and forth. There are some over the counter treatments like gentian violet as well as a miconazole gel that can be compounded by a pharmacy for your baby and the miconazole derm 2% cream that comes with a yeast infection pack. Apply the miconazole derm 2% cream in a thin layer, two to four times daily, for seven days. Make sure you keep going, as if you think it's gone and you stop too soon it will come back. Nystatin is the oldest medicine used for babies to treat thrush, and it has been shown in studies to not be as effective. I will warn you the gentian violet is PURPLE! Really purple and it will not come out; and it will stain your baby's mouth and your breast for a few days. But it really works! Practicing good hygiene while you are treating yourself also keeps thrush from spreading. Wash all towels and bras on hot and let dry in the sun. Consider using disposable paper towels in the bathroom and disposable nursing pads during the treatment. Anything such as toys that your baby puts in their mouth should be sterilized. Please note freezing does not kill yeast so take any pumped milk right to the boiling point or finish up that milk while you are treating the thrush.

It hurts every time my baby latches on and my nipples are cracked and bleeding: Normal or Needs Attention?

Believe it or not I get women in all the time with cracked and bleeding nipples who were told that it's just painful and you have to toughen your nipples up. UM NO! Nursing your baby does have a sensation, but it should not be painful and cause bleeding. Imagine I was blow drying my hair and and I called you and said," My scalp is cracked and bleeding and I'm stomping my feet and wincing everytime this hair dryer starts blowing… You would say NOT NORMAL and let's check out your hair dryer cause that thing must have a busted heating element or something! You will feel a tugging sensation and some suction when nursing but it's not pain. If you feeling pain the first thing to check is your latch. More on that in the next chapter but make sure your baby has a wide open mouth, like a lion plus a little bit. Then when your baby is latched on, use your hand on his shoulder blades to push him in close to you and use the elbow of that same hand like you are scooping ice cream to snuggle his bottom against you. This will make sure the breast is deep in his mouth. Cracked and bleeding nipples always need attention! Find an IBCLC before it gets worse. After you correct the problem you still might feel a three second pain from the prior damage right when your baby latches on but then it will go away and your nipples will get better and better with each feed and not get worse when you are using correct positioning.

My newborn sleeps all the time and won't wake up to nurse: Normal or Needs Attention?

Needs attention! Babies need to eat early and often in the newborn period. First, are you taking any narcotic pain meds? These can make babies sleepy! I am not saying be in pain, I am just saying try to stay away from the narcotic pain medicine or try taking a half of a half and see how little you can use to get by. Another reason besides making your baby sleepy for avoiding narcotic pain medicine is they completely numb you. So you don't feel anything. So picking up that gallon jug of milk from the top shelf in the fridge seems like no big deal, till the medicine wears off and you feel like you've been punched in the stomach. When you are just on the ibuprofen you start to reach for the gallon of milk, and then think, no I should not be lifting that. Don't even get me started on the car seat!!! That thing is soooo heavy! It's called CAR SEAT not easy infant carrier. You can carry a ten pound baby or a nineteen pound car seat. And before you think that car seat can't be nineteen pounds, I just looked it up on Amazon, and the Britax infant car seat says nineteen pounds add a ten pound baby and now you have got twenty-nine pounds! My stomach muscles are hurting just thinking of that. Ok, the car seat rant is over, back to your sleepy baby. In the early weeks babies need to nurse every two hours during the day and every three hours at night with one four hour stretch in twenty-four hours. The easiest way to wake a sleepy baby is called flat surface. Lay your baby on a hard flat surface, the counter, the floor, the glass coffee table. Use just a thin blanket under them and when they feel all the pressure points on their spine then they will start to perk up. Remember they have been floating upside down in a bag full of water for nine months so feeling the pressure of their body is all new to them. You can use your hands like you are petting a puppy to stroke down from the tops of their hips through their legs to get them out of the curled up fetal position and stretch their legs out. Just wait till they are smacking their lips or opening their eyes. You just want to wake them up, not make them mad. Another baby waking technique if your baby falls asleep nursing I call pumping the gas. Take your baby's arm that is towards the ceiling, when your baby is in the nursing position on their side. Hold their hand and lift it up extending it like they are in Pre-Cal saying I know the answer. Their elbow should be straight. Move their hand back towards their shoulder and then reach up again, straightening their elbow, like they are reaching for a gas pump and putting it in the gas tank.

This will usually get them to start sucking again at the breast. You can also talk to them, massage their temple. Rub their hair or lack of hair. Try and see what works best for your baby!

Chapter Three:
Getting started/
What you can really expect

My doula and midwife friends would be miffed if I did not have a little blurb about birth. If you're reading this and you're pregnant please know that having an alert and active childbirth really makes for a great start for breastfeeding. There are some things you can do. Hire a doula; you can do a google search on doulas in your area. You can find more about this in the websites/links and research section in the back of the book. I suggest interviewing one or two that look good and see how you fit. If you are having a home birth with a midwife you probably don't need a doula as your midwife will give you the best personalized care and be your doula midwife all in one!

The most important thing to remember is right after your baby is born, do skin to skin for two hours! This is important and fixes a lot of newborn issues like temperature control. If your baby is cold putting them skin to skin with a warm blanket over both of you has been shown to warm them quicker and keep their temperature more stable than a baby warmer machine. Also, babies skin to skin have been shown to have better oxygen levels and heart rates. When they are skin to skin this also helps them do the breast crawl and latch on themselves. Remember we are mammals! Mama Golden Retriever just lays back after the birth and lets the pups attach. Sure, she adds some licking and cleaning, but all mammals including babies are born with the skills to self attach after birth. The more natural your birth was the easier this is for a baby to do. Do a YouTube search for breast crawl and you will get LOTS of videos of this happening. After the first two hours or so after birth your baby will want to go into a deep sleep. This is why it is so important to meet this person right away and get some nursing in before everyone gets too tired. When the placenta detaches from the uterus this is your body's signal to say, This baby is out of here and needs some milk, let's get this milk making thing going! If you also add to this signal nipple stimulation from your baby nursing, or if your baby is unable to nurse right away hand express some colostrum into a spoon, then you send a double signal to your body, restaurant open for business, let's make some milk! If you already have had your baby and it was a train wreck of a birth read on.

The way to solve many problems is frequent nursing. Frequent nursing helps your milk to come in. I know it may sound like reverse logic, and I said it before, but the emptier your breasts are the faster you're making milk, and the fuller your breasts are the slower you're making milk. Your baby may lose weight from their birth weight, and this seems to freak everyone out, especially when they put it into percentages when they tell it to you. For example, my baby lost ten percent of his birth weight. If your baby weighed seven pounds at birth ten percent of his body weight is 11 oz. This is the time to check into your positioning and make sure your baby is actually drinking at the breast and not just nibbling. There is nothing wrong with your baby nibbling, or comfort nursing, but if that is ALL they do and they are not drinking then that's not going to empty your breasts. The important thing to look at is if this is even "weight" loss or not. If you had IV fluids during labor, and if you had an epidural then you had at least two bags and your baby also had that fluid. So they are born like a juicy Butterball turkey. If you had a boy, and they weighed him all that air on his penis caused him to pee right afterwards. He just lost some fluid. Losing excess fluid or diuresing is normal because all that fluid was EXTRA. The signs of this are a ton of wet and soiled diapers and low numbers on the scale. True weight loss is a lower number on the scale and very few wet and soiled diapers. Remember, your baby needs to have one wet and one soiled diaper per day of life till day 5. So on day 1 its one wet and one soiled, day 2 is two wet and one soiled. Remember this is a twenty-four hour day so if your baby was born at 3 pm you have till 3 pm next day to make your diaper count. So frequent nursing solves many things. It DOES NOT cause sore nipples! You and I could be on a plane right now, in first class (of course) to Maui. And we have huge seats and a comfy pillow to nurse our babies and they stay latched for the seven hour flight. We just sit back and relax and recline in our seats and enjoy the in flight movie and snacks. We arrive in Maui with the same intact nipples that we left with. In contrast, and probably more likely, you and I are on a Southwest Airlines thirty minute flight from Austin to Houston. We are not sitting together because the plane was packed to the gills and we both have middle seats. We are latching on all hunched over with our head under the baby blanket holding our baby at an odd angle. After the thirty minute flight we have a sore nipple that lasts for three days DUE TO POSITIONING! Duration of nursing does not cause sore nipples; it is positioning! If you are using a great position then someone, I suggest a Pediatric Dentist who knows what normal tongue movement and function looks like, should check into your baby's mouth and make sure everything is normal. See tongue tie in next chapter. Another myth of breastfeeding is that it makes babies tired and it burns calories! When everything is normal with your baby's anatomy this is not true! In a study of premature babies the babies who were nursing had better oxygen and slower heart rate than bottle fed babies. When your baby is nursing, and he needs to take a break he just stops, and breathes, and takes a tiny nap and then gets back to it. When your baby is bottle feeding they have to keep swallowing as the milk keeps coming. Now it's time to have some fun with bottles. Take a baby bottle and turn it upside down, it drips, no sucking needed. So your baby has to keep swallowing. Their eyes get really big, and they start swallowing faster and everyone says look, they are gobbling down this bottle, they are so hungry! No, they are protecting their airway! Again, this is just like beer bonging! If you stop swallowing with the hose in your mouth you will drown, that is what regular bottle feeding is. If you are going to feed your baby a bottle. I suggest waiting till your baby is at least six weeks old. Then they know how to nurse and your milk supply is established. You can find more about Paced Bottle Feeding in the websites/links and research section in the back of the book. This is a great way to bottle feed a baby as it allows the flow to be slow and the baby to latch on to the bottle rather than the bottle being put into their mouth, and it allows for breaks, so you baby is less likely to eat so fast that they don't even realize they have eaten. Babies nurse for all kinds of reasons only one of which is hunger. If they are too hot or too cold, nursing fixes that. In a study of twins where they had temp readers on each breast and each twin, if a twin was warmer, the breast surface temp was cooler. The twin that had a cooler temp had a warmer breast temperature. Amazing! If your baby is overstimulated or under stimulated, nursing fixes that! If your baby needs to poop, nursing fixes that. If your baby needs to burp, switching sides or simply pulling them in close to you has gotten a many a baby to burp. Generally, if a baby is under six weeks, try nursing first. If nursing does not work, check their diaper, and try nursing again. If that doesn't work feel their hands, feet, and head, and see if they are too hot or cold. Cover or uncover the body part that is too hot or too cold and then try nursing again. Are you seeing a trend here? Nursing fixes a bunch of problems.

We touched on weight gain earlier, buts let's dive in a little deeper. The best way to tell if your baby is getting enough milk or not is to count their diapers. Six to ten wet diapers and two to four soiled in twenty-four hours is the range. Of course, this is a baby who is over one week. If your baby is having the normal range of diapers, and they are not spending more than half of their day crying, and they are gaining weight, then everything is great! Breastfed babies gain 4 oz to 8 oz a week. The reason this is a range is that the milk has different calorie counts. The milk you make in the morning has different calorie count than what you make in the evening, the milk you make in the middle of the night is different too. This is why it is so important to feed your baby at night. I have had two babies in my practice whose Moms got the advice: "Your baby is six weeks old, and now they don't need to eat at night." Both of these babies had dramatic weight loss! They were swaddled with a pacifier and just sucked on zero calories all night. After a few days of this the Moms, who were engorged during the night when this first started, had lowered their milk supply. So their baby had a lower supply during the day. Lets just be clear. BABIES NEED TO EAT AT NIGHT! The easiest way to accomplish this is by sleeping and nursing at the same time. Before you start to freak out, and say that's not safe let me remind you that there is NO RESEARCH that says co-sleeping with your baby is not safe. The ONE study that showed this was very flawed. It was done by the Consumer Product Safety Commission, and when they looked at the babies who died of co-sleeping they included low birth weight babies, Moms and Dads who were under the influence of drugs and alcohol while sleeping with their baby, and all kinds of other factors that are not safe. You can read all the details about how this study was flawed and find out more about this in the websites/links and research section in the back of the book. So sleeping with your baby is safe if you follow the rules: NEVER sleep on the sofa, the sofa is too squishy and has too many crevices. Don't sleep with your baby if you have had any narcotic pain medicines including cough syrups, or any alcohol or recreational drugs. All of these numb your ability to understand where you are in space when you are asleep and be aware of your surroundings. Keep your baby within arm's reach, his arm's reach not yours. Don't co-sleep with animals in the bed or other children without an adult in between the children. Only co-sleep if you don't smoke and live in a smoke free environment. Keep the bundling to a minimum, your baby will have you as the perfect heater or cooler. Dress your baby as you would dress yourself. Most Moms will curl around on their side in a protective "C" posture. After your baby is moving, make sure you don't have space between the wall and the bed where he can become stuck. Using a bed rail with mesh is a good option as he won't fall through the mesh. Another option is the sidecar arrangement. This is where you take the side off of the crib or drop the side to the lowest setting and put it flush up against the side of your mattress. Finally, you can also get an Arms Reach Co-Sleeper to put your baby in right next to you. I find that the co-sleeper and the sidecar work better because they are the same height as the bed. You can scoot away from your baby slightly and go back to sleep rather than trying to put him down and have him startle and wake up again. The less moving, changing, and talking you do from 11 pm to 5 am the better! You want to send the message that nighttime is for sleeping and nursing, and your baby is not missing out on anything. My oldest was a major sleep fighter. As an infant he would hear a tiny sound and be wide awake, but he grew into a toddler who was sound asleep as we crossed in front of a brass band trying to escape a Disney park during a parade! So just saying, don't worry if you have a sleep issue in a certain stage it is not going to last forever!

At the start I said that I was not going to sugar coat this for you. The reality is that babies NEED people. What most people will not tell you, or they tell you with a tone that says, this is a problem is that babies need to be held most of the time. I'm talking twenty-two out of twenty-four hours. This is really normal and not a problem to be solved. Your babies are born with baby caveman brain; that means when they do not see you or smell you, you do not exist to them. Here is a fun experiment. Take a five month old and show him a toy, a rattle or stuffed animal or anything he wants to grab and then put in his mouth, since that is what five month olds do with anything they are holding. If you are playing with a five month old and shake a toy in front of them, and as he is reaching for it, put it under a blanket, RIGHT IN FRONT OF HIM. He will look at you like, "hey!" His brain does not understand the item exists when he cannot see it. So when you put your baby down and walk into the kitchen, you might as well be on a Caribbean cruise to them. It is only the six month old or older baby that can know you exist when you are out of sight. These babies will lift or drag the blanket to find the item under it that they cannot see. So in your baby's mind if he is alone and cannot see or smell you, he thinks the saber tooth tiger is going to cruise thru the room and eat him. This is a survival instinct all mammals have. Mammal babies call to their Moms to say: 'I'm here, where are you, protect me!'

It is not a bad thing, nor are you creating a crying habit. You are teaching them one of the most important things! Their needs are important. They matter. You are trustworthy, and you will help them. Every single time your baby cries they wonder what will happen even though you have answered their cry ten times in the past four hours. Many Moms notice that when they answer their babies quickly they just make noises instead of crying because their needs are met so quickly. They don't need to full on cry to get what they want. Research shows babies whose cries are responded to in the first six months of life cry less in the next six months of life than the babies who were not responded to as quickly. On the other end of the spectrum, a baby who cries in your arms and does not quiet, knows, on some level, that you are there. They can see you and smell you and they know you are trying to figure it out. The more time you spend with them the more you are able to figure this out. This skill of reading non verbal communication is a skill that will serve you well in the teen years. This is when just like being a newborn, there are few words and you have to decode the mood and emotional health by body posture, eye contact, and other hints that are NOT "Mom, the teacher is really stressing me out!" This is what the first year is like- lots of facial expression reading with not a lot of word communication! Using a baby carrier allows you to do this and have your hands free. Many cities have a babywearing group, where you can try on, and check out all the different baby carriers and find which ones work for you. It's like someone trying to suggest jeans to someone else. These jeans may fit amazing on me, but they just don't work on you. Keep trying different carriers. There is a fit for you out there. Some husbands use their wife's carrier just fine but others like a completely different brand. There are literally tons of videos online on how to wear them.

So if you are still reading and are still tracking with me, you might think this is starting to sound like an Attachment Parenting book. I don't mean it to. However, I have found along with other Moms, this is the easier way. I have had soooo many Moms spend HOURS trying to nurse their babies to sleep, then they lay them down in the crib. The baby wakes up, then they start all over and no one gets to sleep. Or they spend hours trying to put their baby down for a nap, so they can get stuff done, and it takes them several hours of trying, and they never can get the baby down. They don't get to nap, and they get nothing done. Contrast that to this easier way I described when you are sleeping with your baby, and he wakes up and you latch them on and go back to sleep. Your husband never even wakes up at all, and you just wake up for a second. You can wear your baby around in the sling getting what you need done, and they can either nap or not. You get stuff done, and then you take them out of the carrier and nap with them. You also get a nap. So I would not say at all that this is the only way; it's just an easier way. But since I mentioned getting stuff done, know you ARE doing something when you are nursing a baby! Brain development, nutrition, bonding, communication all are happening with breastfeeding. You can listen to a book on Audible, or watch an entire season on Netflix as your baby sleeps, but if your baby is awake then PLEASE talk to him, make eye contact, be present; it's like you being out to dinner with Brad Pitt, and he's on his phone the whole time!! Another idea that seems to be popular right now is having Dad get up to give the baby a bottle at night so Mom can "rest". Now Dad's awake and up feeding the baby, Mom is up pumping because her breasts are used to making milk every two to three hours, and she is too full to be able to sleep for more than three hours, so she is up too. No one is sleeping! Another way is people try and pump before they go to bed, but then you still wake up in three to four hours and have overfull breasts that need to be pumped. So now you are increasing your milk supply, and you are taking out more milk, the timing of the feed is off. I believe the best night is the night where everyone is sleeping. Getting your baby when they are in the early hunger cue phase has him latched on before he even wakes up. He starts nursing and goes back to sleep. There is no need for a diaper change in the middle of the night if you are using disposables if they just pee, unless they seem bothered by it. The disposable diapers seem to lock and load everything, and it will only be three to four more hours before they will be awake again. Having two nursings in a row without changing their diaper for most babies will not be a big problem and lets everyone sleep. Imagine this scenario: you are thirsty in the middle of the night, so you get up, put on your robe and slippers and go downstairs. You get a glass, fill it up with water. You drink it and notice no one started the dishwasher, so you put your glass in and add the soap and turn it on. You go back upstairs, and get into bed. UM, now you are up and it is going to take you fifteen to twenty minutes or more to settle back to sleep. If you're at my house then your husband is also up asking if you are OK, and the dogs are now up and want to go out. Contrast this to having a glass of water next to your bed with a bendy straw, you get up onto your elbow, sip, and lay back down to sleep, and are back to sleep in less than five minutes. The point of this is if your baby is in another room, and you hear him on the monitor, and go get him, change his diaper, and nurse him, he is now UP! It is going to take some settling to get him back to sleep and get you back to sleep. Some Moms have babies who start out in the crib in their room, and the Mom will get them when they wake to nurse, and then bring them into her bed for the rest of the night. If you are thinking well what about some boom boom time with the husband. I say get creative! The guest room? The sofa? It is not like your newborn is going to walk into the living room and start asking you questions! This is the season for boom boom in other rooms of the house, and if you are quiet you might get away with them on the other side of the bed. Soon, you are going to have a crawler, who turns into a walker, and you can't take your eye off him for a second. You are going to take joy in the time when you could put him down and he stayed in the same position you left him in. Moms of nursing toddlers will tell you if they were not nursing they would not sit down all day...at all! Before you freak out that I said nursing a toddler let me have you take a deep breath. I think any day of nursing is a great day. So if you only nurse one day, that's better than zero days. That said this is a relationship, so like any relationship you don't want to end with a bad break up. Ideally, babies nurse until they outgrow the need. Another no one ever told me was the immunities and nutrition of breastmilk are still as strong in a toddler as a newborn. The milk you make for a toddler changes to be exactly what that age toddler needs for growth. The less your toddler nurses the more concentrated the immunities get. So the newborn nursing ten to twelve times a day is getting the same amount of immunities as the toddler nursing four or five times a day; it is just more concentrated. Since nursing toddlers is not the focus of this book I can suggest a great book: "Mothering Your Nursing Toddler" by Norma Jane Bumgarner covers everything you would ever need to know! But wait to think about that until your nursing baby is over one year!

Another thing you can do to prepare is make a plan for food! You must eat breakfast, lunch, and dinner! You don't need to eat extra calories or anything special to make milk but you do not want to skip meals or be hungry! Eating a wide variety of foods as close to their natural state as possible is just sound and normal advice. When you skip meals your blood sugar gets low. If you are reading this before your baby comes then try and make two of whatever you are making and freeze one. It is not really that much more time to make two pans of lasagna at the same time. A popular thing when I was pregnant with my second child was to have a food shower. This is where everyone brings something to freeze with the directions on how to bake or microwave it on the top, instead of gifts. The person hosting can also send out recipes to the guests if you are picky or have diet restrictions. If you have already had your baby then when someone asks how they can help say, bring food! Uber Eats, Postmates or whatever food delivery service is in your area is also a good option. If you are in an area without any options, try pizza delivery, it's better than nothing! Ask for gift cards for food delivery at your baby shower. If you have had your own Mom or your Mother in law in town cooking, and now they are leaving, or your husband has been helping, and is now going back to work, plan now! They can prep some meals for you to have during the day. Hard boiled eggs, already peeled, premade sandwiches, and cut up fruits and veggies, smoothie fixings prepped in a cup in the fridge ready to dump in the blender, are all easy to eat with the one hand you have free while you are nursing.

This is not an exhaustive list of things to do to get a good start. However, I think sleeping and eating are the ones that get the most questions. They are the most important to make sure that you're working on. If you're sleeping and you're eating, things are going to look better even if they're not 100% better. When you're not sleeping and you're not eating the littlest thing can seem like a big deal. After you have a baby you are downloading a whole lot of hormones. Then you add in a low blood sugar, and you get weepy. This goes for toddlers, teens and new Moms. Let any of these people get hungry and tired and you have a mess on your hands. When a Mom calls me for help and is crying on the phone, the first thing I ask her is, "What have you eaten today?" Usually she'll say "some crackers." This is said in between sobs. This is also at 4 o'clock or 5 o'clock in the evening! So then I ask to have her husband put on the phone. I say to her husband, "Go to the fridge, open it up, and tell me what you see." On the most recent call the dad said," I've got some meatloaf…" I said, "Great! Do you have bread?" He said, " yes.." I said," Great. Do you have mayonnaise, lettuce and tomato?" He said, "I have mayonnaise and lettuce…" I said, "Great". He made a meatloaf lettuce mayonnaise sandwich. After his wife had four bites of it she stopped crying, and she was able to calmly talk and tell me what the problem was and how I could help. Happy blood sugar, Happy Mama. If you start to feel weepy, get some food in you! You don't have to eat breakfast food for breakfast and dinner for dinner! If you want oatmeal at 2 pm, eat the oatmeal!

There are a few things you can do to keep yourself out of baby blues land.

These are super important if you have a history of depression, but I think they are good for every new mom. The first one we already covered, but it is so important I will say it again:
Eat breakfast, lunch and dinner.
Take a nap every day; two is even better.

Get some sunshine every day, even if it means just sitting in a sunny window.
Take a shower every day. Even if it means you only have time to shave one leg. Ask me how I know this.
Find a group of Mamas for some support and some fun.

Finally, plan ahead! In your free and single life before kids you could just think about what you wanted to eat right before you ate it. If you were out of a key ingredient you just hopped in the car and got it. Now, hopping in the car is going to take some practice. So look about two hours ahead of the meal. The night before think about breakfast. Can you put some grain in the crock pot with some apples? Do you have all the fixings for breakfast tacos? After breakfast think about lunch. Do you need to defrost anything, soak anything? Can you pop something in the Instant Pot, turn it on and keep it on warm till lunch? This may seem like too much advance planning, compared to before baby but it will really help keep you out of a last minute mental state of hungry, angry, and tired. Once you get in that state it's time to call for help!

Chapter Four:
Overcoming & Troubleshooting

Here are some of the most popular questions I get:

I have a plugged duct! Help!

A plugged duct is just what it sounds like. Imagine there is a pea in your smoothie straw. Well that's what a glob of milk in one of your milk ducts is like. The first thing to notice is its location to imagine how it got there. Here are some places:

On the top of the breast: Are you doing breast compressions too much? On the outer side under your arm: Is the seam on your bra too tight? Underneath your breast: Is your bra the right size? The best way to know if you are in the right size bra or not is to put it on for two hours or so, then take it off and look in the mirror. If you see any compression stripes from where the bra used to be then it's not the right size. This is the same with jeans! Have you ever put on jeans that are too small, and then taken them off only to find that they leave a line down the side of your leg and you can see the zipper print on your belly? The next thing is to check if you are wearing a tank with a shelf bra, make sure you are pulling it down under your breast and not lifting it up and resting on the top of your breast. The pressure of a tight top, bathing suit, or elastic band from a shelf bra can block a duct like pinching a straw shut.

Now that we know what a plugged duct is. Here is how to get rid of it. First, take three Advil. This is over the counter medicine so I am not prescribing you anything. The Advil is an anti inflammatory; it also dilates your milk ducts, allowing the plug to pass through easier. The timing of all this is important. Take the Advil then wait fifteen to twenty minutes and get into a hot bath. If you have a c-section, or your house just does not have a tub, you can do this with a deep pot of hot water. Hot as in hot tub or facial hot, not hot enough to burn you. The important part is that you can submerge your breast in it. When it is submerged, make an E, in sign language with your hand. You can Google how to do that, or you can do it by making a fist and moving your thumb down to be flat against your palm, now the pads of your fingers should be behind the big knuckles on the other side of your hand, and your middle knuckles should be up. With these middle knuckles start with the top of your collar bone and massage straight down towards your nipple, then move your hand over an inch and stroke straight down to your nipple. This is kinda like drawing rays of a sun while your breast is still under water. As you start to get this going you will see a stream of milk come into the water. The milk around the plug is of higher sodium content than regular milk, so it's going to look like smoke in the water coming out of your nipple. Keep on with the radial massage until the stream coming out is clear, not cloudy looking. Then get out of the tub and have your baby nurse or do fifteen minutes of pumping if your baby will not nurse. The baby will always do a better job than the pump, so try to nurse and only use the pump as a last resort. Usually, this works on the first try but it can take two or three times if it is really persistent. The main thing to remember is DO NOT PULL or PICK at the milk strand coming out of your nipple. You will most likely not get it all, and break off some in there, and that can get infected. This goes without saying but never take a needle or anything sharp to your breast. Before you think, no one would do that; trust me, there have been Moms who have done that. It's never pretty!

Another question that I often get: Is it possible to breastfeed when you've had breast surgery?

There are many books on this topic, so I'll just give you the quick and easy answer. Yes, it is possible to breastfeed after breast surgery. The longer amount of time it's been since you had the surgery done the better it goes. Women who have had surgery two years ago and longer usually don't see problems. I've had several women who have had breast surgery who end up having an oversupply of milk! Your breast develops with every period you have from your first one to your last one... you have duct development of your breast. In the beginning when you start your period and during your fertility years you have breast development of the ducts, that's why your breast hurts when it's about time for you to start your period. Toward the end of your periods, when you're nearing menopause, your breast stops making more ducts but starts involuting or does some slight decreasing in tissue so you are not a ninety-year-old woman with Pamela Anderson size breasts. Your muscles just simply can not hold up that much breast at that age. So let's say it's been five years since you have had an implant or breast reduction surgery. In five years you have had sixty periods for your breast to fuse any ducts back together and to build new ducts! So the short answer is, YES! If you need detailed info check out the book, "Defining your Own Success: Breastfeeding After Breast Reduction Surgery" by Diane West.

My baby takes so long to nurse and /or nurses all the time.

This is a common concern where people think something is wrong, or they want nursing to be quicker. The average baby takes about thirty minutes to take in about 2.0 oz. This is average, the middle, or for all you math nerds out there, the median. There are some babies who are much quicker. They nurse in about three or four minutes. They are usually older, say six months or more or, if they are younger and you have an oversupply of milk. You've read about oversupply earlier. Then there is the other side of the median where you have a normal anatomy baby and Mom, with a normal milk supply who nurses for forty minutes. This can also be normal. Things to consider to decide if this is an issue or if this is just your baby's eating type. Yes, I said eating type. We all have an eating type. If we all went to dinner right now, and ordered at the same time we would all finish at different times. My husband and I, having fussy babies and being on call would eat and finish in ten minutes or less. Really. You might be super chatty and only be a few bites into your meal. Your design focused friend might be taking in the décor of the restaurant and have not even started on her meal. All of us are normal. We just have different eating types. Some babies are snackers. Some are super efficient. Others are more leisure eaters who take breaks. All of these can be normal if your wet and soiled diaper count is normal, if your baby spends most of his day happy, or if he is gaining well and his growth is on an upward curve. This might be a good time to bring up growth charts. There are growth charts by the World Health Organization available online for boys and girls who are breastfed and from a variety of cultures. Most pediatrician offices still use the growth charts that were based on formula fed babies from the same ethnic group (white) from the 50's. So if you are Italian or Asian and the tallest person in your family is 5'5" then your baby is going to be low or maybe in the one percentile on this chart. I urge you to not get stressed out about what percentile your baby is in but rather if they are continuing to grow in an upward curve for their gender and age. Exclusively breastfed babies grow in a different way than formula fed babies. You cannot overfeed a breastfed baby as the milk changes in calorie count from time of the day to age of baby. So it's possible for your breastfed baby to gain the average of one oz a day or they could gain a little different each day. Something like: on Monday, not lose weight but not gain, then gain 2 oz on Tuesday, then .5 oz on Wednesday, then gain 3 oz on Thurs, not gain or lose on

Friday, and gain 1 oz on Sat. In total that is 6.5 oz gain in a week. This is well within the normal range of 4 oz to 8 oz a week. Formula, in contrast, is the same calorie count. This is not a mystery, just look on the back of the can and it tells you how many calories there are. It tastes exactly the same each time and has exactly the same calories each time. So if you are just thirsty, you get a big burger, a little hungry, a big burger, really, really, hungry, a big burger, really just tired and needing some comfort, you guessed it, big burger. I am not slamming formula here. If you don't have any pumped milk, and you don't have a Milk Bank in your area and cannot get milk from another Mother then formula is an option. But it is a tool to make breastfeeding work not a solution. Think of it as duct tape. You can tape a hose of your car engine together to get you to the mechanic but you would not want to drive the car forever with the tape on it, you would want to get it fixed.

My baby is jaundiced and they want to give him formula!

Once in a while I get a call from a Mom who has a jaundiced baby. The simplest explanation of jaundice is not getting the bilirubin out by pooping, which is actually your baby pooping out the red blood cells to break them down. For most babies this is not a problem and a slight yellow color that goes from their head gradually down their trunk, then disappears back up their trunk again, is the progression of their body processing the extra red blood cells that they needed in the womb and do not need anymore. No need to worry if your baby is doing plenty of nursing, has plenty of wet and soiled diapers, and is waking up easily to nurse. Nursing in a sunny spot with your baby dressed in only a diaper may be helpful. The main thing to do for jaundice is nurse. You can hand express a little after each feed, or pump if your milk is in and give them even more of your milk with a syringe, cup, or spoon. The thing you do not want to do is give formula or anything but breastmilk. This will be harder to poo out, making them constipated, and not getting the bilirubin out. The slight yellow color is just what babies go through to get rid of the red blood cells that they don't need anymore. If the bilirubin levels are high, then you can request a bili blanket sent to your house in four hours by the company, My Bili Blanket, as long as you have a prescription from your pediatrician. You can find more about this in the websites/links and research section in the back of the book. One Mom, who did not live in the delivery area for a bili blanket, said her children's hospital put her in a bikini top and had her hold her baby while sitting under the bili lights and nurse him at the hospital, instead of putting baby under bili lights by himself. I really like this as it keeps Mom and baby together and gives light therapy at the same time. I also like Dr. Jack Newman's explanation of jaundice. You can find more about this in the websites/links and research section in the back of the book. In short, plenty of nursing, make sure you're getting plenty of wet and soiled diapers and ask for a bili blanket if you need more help.

Oversupply and overactive let down

Some Moms make a ton of milk. All the Moms who don't make a ton of milk think this would be an amazing problem to have, but let me assure you it comes with its own drawbacks. When your baby just wants a snack they get the full meal deal, fast! Some things you can do to slow the flow are: use a laid back position. Try and get the line from your shoulder to your hip at a ninety degree angle. This is easier when you lean against the side arm of a sofa with your legs across the sofa. This makes the milk go up hill from your breast to your baby instead of the milk working with gravity, when you lean over your baby. Short frequent feeds also keep your breast comfortable while leaving milk in the breast. When milk is left in the breast it is a signal to your body to make less milk the next time. This also keeps your breast from getting too full or engorged. Pumping, in contrast completely empties your breast. While this may sound and feel heavenly, it is short lived. Now you have just sent the signal to rev up the supply even more and in the next two hours your breasts are going to be even fuller. If the baby is not taking what you need to be comfortable, first try encouraging your baby to nurse more. If that is not working then pump for two to three minutes just until you feel full but no longer feel hot, heavy and tight. It's not going to give you immediate relief but will help you to tell your body to make less milk at the next feed and with each feed you will feel better and better. If this is not working another thing to try is some cabbage. I know, it sounds crazy but there is an enzyme in green cabbage that reacts with your skin to make your milk supply decrease. We talked about how to use it in the earlier chapter on normal vs needs attention. But you're a new Mom so I will give you a recap rather than have you flip back. Take the leaves of the cabbage and wrap your breast in them. Imagine you are making a mummy costume with the cabbage and cover all sides, then nipple and the top with the leaves. Then put your bra flaps up to hold all of this in place. Cue the Oktoberfest music and put on the corned beef! Seriously, let the cabbage wilt till it looks like cooked cabbage. If you can put your fingernail in it and it still has a crunch to it, it has not been on long enough, you need about two hours or so. For some women this can be very effective and strong. I have heard from other IBCLC's that using it too much too often has dried up women's milk. I have never personally seen this but I think if you slept in the cabbage, did it multiple times a day, or your milk supply wasn't that high to begin with then it is possible. Remember to set an alarm if you are using it and taking a nap to avoid overdoing it.

Weight gain or lack of weight gain is another issue people have right from the start.

We have touched all over it in different places but here it is in a nutshell. The way to tell how much a baby is getting is diapers, how your baby seems (are they screaming most of the day), and lastly numbers on the scale. What comes in must come out. If you are on one of those Survivor reality shows where all you have to eat one day is a bug you are not going to poo three times that day! Marginal gain equals marginal poo and needs to get some attention. If you're not having six to ten wet and two to four soiled diapers in twenty-four hours, your baby may not be getting enough.

The next thing to do is find an IBCLC who can weigh your baby, then have you nurse your baby then weigh your baby. When your baby is at least one week old you can use the mathematical equation of babies weight in pounds multiplied by 2.0 to 2.5 oz equals the number of ounces needed in twenty-four hours. So a baby who is 7 lbs x 2.5 oz needs 17.5 oz of milk in twenty-four hours . If you are feeding ten times in twenty-four hours then that's 1.7 oz per feed. From two weeks to six months the calorie count in milk increases so you do not need to increase the amount of the feed. This is only true with breastmilk. Read the back of the can, formula is the same calorie count every time. If your transfer is not 2.0 oz or close you can first just try to increase the amount of time and the quality of nursing. I am telling you this for info, do not obsess over the numbers. I am giving you this info so if someone tells you your baby needs a little extra milk, that amount would be .5 oz, half the feed would be 1.0 oz, and the whole feed is 2.0 oz to 2.5 oz. This equation only works with a baby who is from one week until twelve weeks old. Babies should have about thirty minutes of active sucking at the breast to get the milk they need for the feed. This does not mean the time when they are sleeping, with the breast in their mouth, or doing the suck that feels like butterfly wings fluttering across your nipple. This is active sucking, it's ok for them to have times of light suck but that is assuming they are gaining well and the diaper count is good. For a look at what normal looks like check out Dr. Jack Newman's videos on really good drinking. You can find more about this in the websites/links and research section in the back of the book.

Notice in the video how the cheek is flush with the breast. This is important. Your baby can breathe. If you're worried their nose is too squished then you can push their chin in by pushing on their shoulder blades. This will push their chin in and and nose out. Seeing an IBCLC in person will help you get the best latch possible. I am going to talk you through it but it's pretty visual so hang in there.

First, get comfortable. We are going to just talk about the cradle hold position as it is the easiest to do when you are just starting out. Make sure your feet touch the floor. Make sure your back is supported. I like to use the My Breast Friend Pillow, it's firmer and it buckles around you so it does not slip out and have your baby in a hole on your lap and the nursing pillow behind your baby. The pillow should be right under your breast so when your baby is laying on their side they are being supported by the pillow and at breast height, so they are nose to nipple with their neck being in a neutral position, not reaching up and not reaching down chin to chest. You can put pillows under the nursing pillow or use a stack of bed pillows. You should not have to hunch over and bend down to them, your back should be against the back of the cushion and you should be comfy. Next, draw a line from your nipple diagonally out across your pillow to the edge of the pillow. This line you can make a mental note of, or if you're really sleep deprived you can put a tiny post it note on the edge of the pillow. This is a visual reminder of where your baby is to be lined up with your nipple. If he is four inches higher or lower than your line or post it, then the nipple is twisted in his mouth; it's being sucked on at an angle. It will come out of his mouth in a lipstick shape. This can also be caused at latch on by moving your breast and twisting your nipple toward him. Move the baby not the breast! Your nipples are where they are supposed to be. Scoot your baby's bottom up to get him nose to nipple or hold him under his arms and move him down, towards the breast he is not nursing on to get him lined up. Once he has a wide open mouth, using your hand on his shoulder blades and not on his head, use your elbow as if you are scooping ice cream to bring him tummy to tummy with you. I cannot stress enough to not hold his head like a stick shift in the car. When you grab a baby's head they arch their back, and now he is moving away from you instead of toward the breast. Go back and check out the good drinking links from Dr. Jack Newman to refresh yourself on what that looks like.

Hunger Cues: When is my baby ready to nurse?

The earliest sign your baby is ready to nurse is when he is in REM sleep. You can see his eyeballs moving rapidly under his closed eyes. The next thing that will happen is that he will open his eyes, then he will smack his lips, and stick out his tongue, next he is going to root to anything nearby, then he is going to try and suck anything near, his hand, the side of the car seat, your shoulder. Finally he gets to crying! If you get to crying you have missed steps 1-5 and now he is mad. Crying is a late sign of hunger. The time to get ready is when he is in REM sleep. Grab anything you might need, water, snack, book on tape, remote, pillow, blanket and get comfortable. The next cue is he is going to open his eyes, HI! This is the time to position him to latch, by lining him up nose to nipple, making sure he is at breast height, so your breast is resting on the pillow. If you are large breasted using a washcloth rolled up like a foam roller and placed under your breast can help lift the nipple off the pillow. Next, stroke his lips with the breast going from the top of his lips through his mouth and back up again. This will trigger a reflex for him to open his mouth wide. When he does, come together as if you were going to dance with someone. You would not slam them to you, nor would you hold them at arms length and hesitate. Just come together gradually, use your elbow of the arm holding him to scoop him toward you like you are scooping ice cream with your elbow. Relax your shoulders, talk, sing and coo to your new little one. This is just the cradle hold. The La Leche League website has some great info about all other positions and the website www.mother2mother.com will show you with detailed pictures how to nurse lying down in bed. Mentioning La Leche League has reminded me of our next chapter.

Chapter Five:
How and where to get help

If you are having pain when nursing the first thing to do is contact an International Board Certified Lactation Consultant. Please recall the differences between a CLC and an IBCLC that I presented earlier. You want an IBCLC, remember she is required to have hours of hands on Mom and baby time, and she recertified every five years with continuing education credits and every ten years by exam. If you just have a general breastfeeding question or you want the support of other Moms read on and get yourself to a La Leche League Meeting. LLL Groups meet once a month and many cities have several groups.

 La Leche League (LLL) is non profit, non denominational nursing Mothers organization that started in 1956 with a group of Mothers who were nursing their babies at a picnic in Franklin Park, IL. These women had other women come up to them and say, "I really wanted to nurse my baby but…" and then you insert any crazy myth about breastfeeding in the blank. My doctor said my milk was too thin; it took too much time. My baby did not like it. I don't know what the exact myths were, but the women at the picnic said come to our house. We will talk about breastfeeding. Seven women founded LLL, and now it is in 81 countries worldwide and their book "The Womanly Art of Breastfeeding" is in its 8th edition. LLL today is based on the same concepts as it was back then, women and their babies and toddlers sitting around talking and helping each other with breastfeeding. A long time ago, before air travel everyone lived down the street from each other. When you had a baby your Mom, Aunt and Cousins would come over and help you. They would feed you and show you how to nurse lying down and calm you with stories of nursing you or their own babies, But now people are all spread out over the country, and your own Mom may not have nursed you or even remembered the details. The LLL book, "The Womanly Art of Breastfeeding" is still the most comprehensive book I know about breastfeeding. It is medically referenced in the back, so it's not just someone's opinion, It is based, like this book, on real research. Some fun trivia.   My son Luke is pictured on the loving guidance chapter page in the 6th edition of "The Womanly Art of Breastfeeding"! We were at a LLL conference in Chicago, and he took his first steps there.   All of the founders were alive then, and they all signed the page of his picture. He is also the cover model for this book, which is probably super embarrassing for a teenager but I hope one day when he has a baby of his own, he will find it sweet. Ok, maybe his wife will find it sweet?

I have been an accredited La Leche League Leader since 1998. I continue to lead meetings in Austin, TX because with my

IBCLC work all I see is problems. No one really makes an appointment with me to just chat about babies! I like to see Moms who are nursing their babies and want to share and chat with some other Moms. If all I saw were problems I would forget that a lot of Moms don't have any problems with nursing! There is a myth about LLL that it is only for people with nursing issues. Oddly, people also think it is for people without issues. Let me clear that up, it is for both. You can come to LLL if you need help, just want to talk, or are pregnant and want to know what this nursing thing is all about. The Moms at the meeting just know me as Ann Bennett LLL Leader, not as an IBCLC. In that meeting I am there to clarify LLL philosophy and let Moms have a place to brainstorm with each other how to navigate this time and hear what works for each Mom. Every Mother is an expert on her own baby, and every Mother knows her baby best. When my oldest was small our La Leche League group was HUGE, twenty-five or more Moms in the gym of a church, and we would have potlucks after the meeting and playgroups. Most LLL groups meet in churches or library meeting rooms as they are free. We are non profit. We don't have any money to pay for a space to lease. Each LLL group has its own flavor and that can change each month. So if you find a group near you and you go and it's not your tribe, try another group or that same group another month. Babies and toddlers are always welcome at LLL meetings. Some LLL groups have a separate group for couples but for the most part it's only Moms allowed. The reason for this is simple. Most of theses Moms are nursing for the first time in public, and it's more comfortable to be with all Moms than a mixed group. LLL loves men and thinks they are vital to babies and Mamas!

Tongue tie is another topic Moms often say, "Why did no one mention this?" When your baby is born you are able to check to see if they need to be seen by a professional to evaluate if they have a tongue tie or not.

This is not as complicated as it may seem. When your baby is crying, a diaper change is a great place to check this. Pull down his chin to his chest. I find using your thumb going east to west across his chin and applying gentle pressure works best. Then see if his tongue tip touches the top of the roof of his mouth. To the roof is perfect. Very close is OK, but if the tip of the tongue does not lift past the corners of his mouth, or it lays flat on the floor of his mouth, he needs an evaluation. Remember to do this with a wide open mouth. When the tongue is being tied from the middle or back, it looks like you could put a marble in a tiny depression that forms in the middle of the tongue since it is being pulled from underneath. When the baby latches on to the breast the bottom of his tongue acts like the bottom of a bun, the breast is the burger in the middle, and the roof of the baby's mouth is the top bun. To get milk out of the breast the baby lifts his tongue to the roof, thus squeezing the breast against his soft palate and then the milk comes out. If his tongue does not reach, not only does nothing come out but instead of the tongue going under the breast in a comfortable way, it hits at the nipple causing damage. A great resource with pictures of tongue tie and how to see what it looks like is from Catherine Watts Genna IBCLC, called "Is My Baby Tongue Tied". You can find more about this in the websites/links and research section in the back of the book. Check out the pictures and compare them to your baby. Check this on day one or two of life. The earlier you get this seen the sooner you can correct the problem and thus the shorter the time it will be to regain normal nursing. When your baby cannot use his tongue to nurse correctly it causes cracked and bleeding nipples. It also lowers the milk supply as the baby is leaving milk in the breast. Since the baby is not transferring well you have low weight gain. When you get this corrected on day three to five it seems to reduce all the other problems. Anytime is a good time for a correction. Some Moms don't check this until their baby is two weeks, after trying everything else under the sun, and in a few weeks after getting it fixed they are back on track. As a rule as long as they have been nursing with their tongue incorrectly is about the same time it will take them to figure out how to do it correctly again. So if you are getting it corrected on day seven it takes about another seven days to be completely improved. You will notice a difference right away! But your baby will have function, not stamina and your milk supply may need some support with pumping and an herbal product like More Milk Plus. Remember, every day you are making some improvement! Progress not Perfection!

Now the Who's Who in Tongue Tie! There are many providers who do a frenotomy. Let's unpack this:

The Pediatric Ear Nose and Throat (Pedi ENT): The Pedi ENT sees mostly problems. Like the IBCLC no one makes an appointment with them just to chat and see normal. They do the procedure with a scissor. This does bleed. If the tongue tie is right on the tip sometimes this can work. However, studies have shown that if the type of tongue tie is type four, the back of the tongue, it is too vascular and may not be able to be released completely without a bleed. So with Pedi ENT scissors, and bleeding will occur. It is harder to do on a tie that is located on the back of the tongue. Healing time is longer than with other methods.

The next person is the Pediatric Dentist. Unlike the Pedi ENT the Pedi Dentist sees NORMAL. They see what a one year old tongue looks like and they see what a ten year old tongue looks like. They get kids in for regular cleanings and checkups. The one we have in town has shared some educational pictures with me of before and after of my clients with my clients' approval and it does not bleed as it cauterizes as it goes, since it is all done with a laser. Laser works on the vascular ones as well as the ones at the tip. The healing is much quicker than the scissor as it just takes the lightest layer off and does not get into the muscle.

So to recap the tongue tie issue. When your baby is born, check his tongue for amount of lift with a wide open mouth, his chin pulled down to his chest. If it's not lifting or you are not sure, search in your area for a Pedi Dentist or other provider who uses a laser and read the reviews from others. Calling an IBCLC in your area might also give you some good ideas on who they refer to. Tongue tie can cause low milk supply, low weight gain, and nipple damage and is better addressed early. Many babies go on to have a happy and great nursing relationship after the revision. Think of it as ding in the door of your new car; it may have a door ding, but it still drives great and looks beautiful!

I do want to put a blurb in here about Craniosacral Therapy (CST). Most of the time I am the first person to mention this to a Mom and she has never heard of it. Since you are reading this, that won't be you. CST is a very light massage of your babies cranial nerves, the nerves in the head. Your baby has been upside down in a bag full of water in a tight position and they have been pushed and squeezed via birth and sometimes these nerves can be out of whack and need some TLC. Think of it as Occupational Therapy for your babies mouth since the tongue, jaw, swallowing, and sucking all use these nerves. The person doing CST should be registered and have experience with babies. You can call an IBCLC in your area and ask who they refer to. CST can help with a baby who has had a tongue tie revised, a baby with a tight jaw who has trouble getting a wide latch, and babies who just seem disorganized have trouble getting latched on. Think of it like this, If you and I got in a car wreck and you had a massage every day and I did not, you would feel better sooner. Would we both get better eventually, YES. But you would feel better faster, and have a better range of motion sooner, as all of your tissue and nerves are in the right places to work at their best. CST helps babies to relax and not work so hard. Many Moms report their babies love having CST and say its like going to the day spa for babies.

Sometimes I get a call where a Mom looked up some information online and is now freaking out. The information was usually found between 10pm and 4am. I suggest you don't google anything that you are worried about after 10pm, I'm not joking, you are tired from the day and your mind can go to all sorts of places that it would not go during the daylight.

When you are looking for information some sites are more accurate than others. Anyone can make a web page about anything so making sure you are on a site that is providing you with non sponsored, researched based accurate information is important.

I have a few suggestions for you. First, for general info you can't beat the La Leche

League site mentioned above.
www.LLLi.org

I also like www.Kellymom.com. This site is done by IBCLC's and has the medical referenced resources listed for where the information came from. I really like the tone and it is easy to find stuff and navigate. Kellymom is great for articles on weight gain and jaundice, if you are just having a freak out and need a quick answer, info about how to cure thrush, and lots of other stuff that if we cover in detail here, this book would be too heavy to hold and nurse at the same time!

Another good source for all topics is www.askdrsears.com

I really cannot imagine a question or a topic that you would need to know that is not on one of these sites.

The books that I suggest are:

"The Womanly Art of Breastfeeding" by La Leche League- This book is written in such a warm and easy to read tone. I love all the Mom's stories! Plus you can basically fact check the book as it is medically referenced in the back like my book. We are not making this stuff up people!

"The Baby Book" by Sears- This covers everything you need to know from birth until age two, My copy was so worn that it is coming unbound. I had Dr. Bill and Martha Sears sign it at a conference and they said they wished all their books looked like that. I also hope for the same with this book, throw it in your diaper bag, have it next to your bed, have it in the pocket of your nursing pillow, and pick it up whenever you need a little cheer from me and to be reminded you are doing this! Your experience may not be the same as other Moms, but it is YOUR journey!

Final Thoughts

The new baby time is a season filled with joys and tears. It's about leaning into your baby and leaning away from yourself. But it is just for a time. As I write this, my oldest has just gone back to college in Pittsburgh from being home for Spring break, and my high schooler, who is a junior, is off skiing with friends for his Spring Break with a family who has a house in Colorado. My husband and I are eating at a fancy restaurant that we haven't been to in twenty-three years. When our oldest was born if we could sit in the car at Sonic and have our tots and cheese and cherry limeade without having a screaming baby wake up it was considered a miracle! But here we are, twenty-three years later. I'm telling you this to give you hope. I wish that I could go back and tell this to myself as a Mom when I had a new baby, and I'm crying at the fancy Easter buffet when I'm having to shove food into my mouth as quickly as possible because my husband is walking squirmy screaming baby, who will not sit in his high chair, outside. All I wanted to do then was sit and eat and enjoy my family. Remember that this time is limited. I've come through to the other side and I can look back and tell you it's not always going to be this way. So when you feel like you're a prisoner of nursing and you're having a day when all you're doing is nursing, or you're wondering if you're ever going to be able to eat out at a place that has real silverware again. I want to encourage you to hang in there. I got through this and you will get through this.

So buckle in, bra flaps up, or down if it's time to nurse, and enjoy the good times and the hard times and know that this is temporary, and most importantly remember: I'm rooting for you, and God walks with you.

Websites & Links

Info on cancer prevention from breastfeeding
https://www.mdanderson.org/publications/focused-on-health/october-2014/breastfeeding-breast-cancer-prevention.html

James McKenna Mother baby sleep lap
https://cosleeping.nd.edu

Video on how to do paced bottle feeding
https://www.youtube.com/watch?v=UH4T70OSzGs

To find a doula
https://doulamatch.net/search and here:
http://www.dona.org

How the one sleep study was flawed
https://www.askdrsears.com/topics/health-concerns/sleep-problems/sids-latest-research-how-sleeping-your-baby-safe.

To order a bili blanket
http://mybiliblanket.com/how_to_order

Dr. Jack Newman on Jaundice

https://ibconline.ca/information-sheets/breastfeeding-and-jaundice/

Dr. Jack Newman's videos on good drinking
https://www.breastfeedinginc.ca/videos/really-good-drinking/

Nursing lying down instructions with pictures
www.mother2mother.com

Catherine Watts Genna IBCLC Is my baby tongue tied?
http://www.cwgenna.com/ttidentify.html

Great video on hands on how to get more pumping if your supply is low: Search Standford Maximizing Milk Production

La Leche League www.LLLi.org

Kellymom www.Kellymom.com

Dr Sears www.askdrsears.com

References & Research

Sleeping with your baby and the research on when done correctly it is safe

Baddock SA, Galland BC, Taylor BJ, Bolton DPG 2007, Sleep arrangements and behavior of bed-sharing families in the home setting. *Pediatrics* 119(1): e200–e207.

Ball HL, Hooker E, Kelly PJ 2000, Parent-infant co-sleeping: Fathers' roles and perspectives. *Inf Child Dev* 9: 67–74.

Ball H L 2002, Reasons to bed-share: why parents sleep with their infants. *J Reproduct Infant Psychol* 20 (4): 207-222.

Ball HL 2003, Breastfeeding, bed sharing and infant sleep. *Birth* 30(3): 181–188. Blair PS, Fleming PJ, Smith IJ, Ward Platt M, Young J, Nadin P, Berry PJ, Golding

Blair PS, Heron J, Fleming PH 2010, Relationship between bed sharing and breastfeeding: longitudinal, population-based analysis. *Pediatrics* 126(5): e1119–e1126.

Byard RW, Beal S, Blackbourne B, Nadeau JM, Krous HDF 2001, Specific dangers associated with infants sleeping on sofas. *J Paediatr Child Health* 37: 476–478.

Carpenter RG, Irgens LM, Blair PS, England PD, Fleming P, Huber J, Jorch G,control study. *Lancet* 363: 185–191.

EM, Becroft DMO on behalf of the New Zealand Cot Death Study Group 1993, Bed sharing, smoking, and alcohol in the sudden infant death syndrome. *BMJ* 307:1312–1318.

Hauck FR, Thompson JM, Tanabe KO, Moon RY, Vennemann MM, 2011,Breastfeeding and reduced risk of sudden infant death syndrome: a meta-analysis.*Pediatrics* 128(1):103–110.

J, CESDI SUDI Research Group 1999, Babies sleeping with parents: case-control study of factors influencing the risk of the sudden infant death syndrome. *BMJ* 319: 1457–1461.

McCoy RC, Hunt CE, Lesko SM, Vezina R, Corwin MJ, Willinger M, Ho man HJ,Mitchell AA 2004, Frequency of bed sharing and its relationship to breastfeeding.*Dev Behav Pediatr* 25(3): 141–114.

McKenna JJ, McDade T 2005, Why babies should never sleep alone: a review of the co-sleeping controversy in relation to SIDS, bedsharing and breastfeeding *Paediatr Respir Rev* 6(2): 134–152.

Righard, L. and Alade, M. O. (1997), Breastfeeding and the Use of Pacifiers. Birth, 24: 116-120. doi:10.1111/j.1523-536X.1997.tb00351.x

SIDS and Kids and Queensland Health 2012, *Safe Sleeping Brochure.* URL: *http://sidsandkids.org/ wp-content/uploads/SafeSleeping_Brochure.pdf* Accessed 1/10/12.

UNICEF UK Baby Friendly Initiative 2004, *Babies Sharing Their Mother's Bed While In Hospital A Sample Policy* URL: *http://www.unicef.org.uk/ BabyFriendly/Resources/Guidance-for-Health-Professionals/Writing-policies-and-guidelines/ Sample-bedsharing-policy/* Accessed 1/10/12.

UNICEF UK 2011, *Caring For Your Baby at Night* (Lea et) URL: *http://www.unicef.org.uk/ BabyFriendly/Resources/Resources-for-parents/ Caring-for-your-baby-at-night/* Accessed 1/10/12. Vennemann MM, Hense HW, Bajanowski T, Blair PS, Complojer C, Moon RY et al 2012, Bed sharing and the risk of sudden infant death syndrome: can we resolve the debate? *J Pediatr* 160(1): 44–48.e2.
World Health Organization Child Growth Standards, 2006. Available at: http://www.who.int/childgrowth/en/.

Young J 1998, Bed-sharing with babies: the facts. *RCM Midwives Journal* 1(11): 338–341 Young J 1999, *Night-time Behaviour and Interactions Between Mothers and Their Infants Low Risk for SIDS: A Longitudinal Study of Room-sharing and Bed sharing*, PhD thesis: Institute of Child Health, University of Bristol.

Milk supply

Cregan MD, Hartmann PE. Computerized breast measurement from conception to weaning: clinical implications. J Hum Lact 1999; 15(2):89-96.

Daly SEJ, Hartmann, PE: Infant demand and milk supply. Part 1: Infant demand and milk supply in lactating women. J Hum Lact 1995; 11(1):21-26.

Daly SEJ, Hartmann, PE: Infant demand and milk supply. Part 2: The short-term control of milk synthesis in lactating women. J Hum Lact 1995; 11(1):27-31.

Daly SEJ, Kent JC, Huynh DQ, Owens RA, Alexander BF, Ng, KC, Hartmann PE. The determination of short-term volume changes and the rate of synthesis of human milk using computerized breast measurement. Experimental Physiology 1992; 77:79-87.

Jaundice

Academy of Breastfeeding Medicine Clinical Protocol #22: Guidelines for Management of Jaundice in the Breastfeeding Infant Equal to or Greater Than 35 Weeks' Gestation from *Breastfeeding Medicine* Vol. 5 No. 2; 2010: pp 87-93.

http://pediatrics.aappublications.org/content/114/1/297.full

General References

La Leche League International Web Site,. "The Benefits of Breastfeeding A-Z." and "The Game Normal vs Needs attention". *Leader Pages,* 3 Mar. 2011,

Mohrbacher N and Stock J. The Breastfeeding Answer Book, Third Revised ed. Schaumburg, Illinois: La Leche League International, 2003.

Riordan J. Breastfeeding and Human Lactation, 3rd ed. Boston: Jones and Bartlett, 2005

Wiessinger, Diane., Diana West, Teresa Pitman, and La Leche League International. *The Womanly Art of Breastfeeding.* 8th ed. New York: Ballantine Books, 2010

Studies on how breastmilk is brain food

"Breast milk makes kids brighter, study suggests" – a news article from CNN. This is about the study that was done in New Zealand, based on a review of more than 1,000 children born in New Zealand in 1977 and followed through age 18.

Breastfeeding and Later Cognitive and Academic Outcomes– the actual journal article referenced above (PEDIATRICS Vol. 101 No. 1 January 1998, p. e9).

Lucas A, Morley R, Cole TJ. Randomised trial of early diet in preterm babies and later intelligence quotient. BMJ. 1998 Nov 28;317(7171):1481-7.

Mortensen EL, Michaelsen KF, Sanders SA, Reinisch JM. The Association Between Duration of Breastfeeding and Adult Intelligence. JAMA. 2002;287:2365-2371. "Independent of a wide range of possible confounding factors, a significant positive association between duration of breastfeeding and intelligence was observed in 2 independent samples of young adults, assessed with 2 different intelligence tests."

N K Angelsen, T Vik, G Jacobsen, and L S Bakketeig. Breastfeeding and cognitive development at age 1 and 5 years (abstract). Arch. Dis. Child. 2001; 85: 183-188.

Pregnancy and Nursing May Make Women Smarter. Hormones released during pregnancy and nursing enrich parts of the Mother's brain involved in learning and memory, a study of animals suggests.

Babies do not need Vitamin D supplement

http://staging.llli.org/nb/nbjulaug04p124.html

Barber, K. and Purnell-O'Neal, M. The politics of vitamin D: Questioning universal supplementation. Mothering 2003 Mar-Apr; 117:52-63.
Good Mojab, C. Personal communication, July 2, 2004.

Good Mojab, C. Sunlight deficiency: A review of the literature. Mothering 2003 Mar-Apr; 117:52-63.

Good Mojab, C. What ingredients are in vitamin supplements? Mothering 2003 Mar-Apr; 117:52-63.

Heaney, R.P. et al. Human serum 25-hydroxycholecalciferol response to extended oral dosing with cholecalciferol. Am J Clin Nutr 2003; 77(1):204-10.

Heinig, M.J. Vitamin D and the breastfed infant: Controversies and concerns. J Hum Lact 2003; 19(3).

Nesby-O'Dell, S. et al. Hypovitaminosis D prevalence and determinants among African American and white women of reproductive age. Am J Clin Nutr 2002 Jul; 76(1):3-4.

Shaikh, U. and Alpert, P. Practices of vitamin D recommendation in Las Vegas, Nevada. J Hum Lact 2004; 20(1).

Specker, B. et al. Sunshine exposure and serum 25-hydroxyvitamin D concentrations in exclusively breastfed infants. J Pediatr 1985; 107:372-76.

Breastfeeding lowers risk of obesity

Dewey KG, Heinig MJ, Nommsen LA, Peerson JM, Lonnerdal B. Growth of breast-fed and formula-fed infants from 0 to 18 months: the DARLING Study. Pediatrics 1992 89(6): 1035-1041.

Gillman MW, et al. Risk of overweight among adolescents who were breastfed as infants. JAMA 2001 May 16;285(19):2461-7.

Hediger ML, Overpeck MD, Kuczmarski RJ, Ruan WJ. Association Between Infant Breastfeeding and Overweight in Young Children. JAMA 2001;285:2453-2460.

Koletzko B, von Kries R. Are there long term protective effects of breastfeeding against later obesity? Nutr Health 2001;15(3-4):225-36.

Toschke AM, et al. Overweight and obesity in 6- to 14-year-old Czech children in 1991: protective effect of breast-feeding. J Pediatr 2002 Dec;141(6):764-9.

Von Kries R, Koletzko B, Sauerwald T, von Mutius E. Does breastfeeding protect against childhood obesity? Adv Exp Med Biol 2000;478:29-39.

Von Kries R, et al. Breastfeeding and obesity: cross sectional study. BMJ 1999 Jul 17;319(7203):147-50.

Studies on how breastfeeding protects against cancer

Breastfeeding may protect against some forms of childhood leukemia. The new study, by researchers in Israel (published in JAMA Pediatrics), found that 14% to 20% of all childhood leukemia cases may be prevented by breastfeeding for 6 months or more. [Efrat L. Amitay, PhD, MPH; Lital Keinan-Boker, MD, PhD, MPH. Breastfeeding and Childhood Leukemia Incidence *JAMA Pediatr*. 2015;169(6):e151025]

HAMLET kills tumor cells by an apoptosis-like mechanism. The acid pH in the stomach of the breast-fed child \promotes the formation of HAMLET. This mechanism may contribute to the protective effect of breastfeeding against childhood tumors. [Svanborg C, Agerstam H, et al. *Adv Cancer Res*. 2003;88:1-29.]

Tongue Tie Research

Buryk, M., Bloom, D., & Shope, T. (2011). Efficacy of neonatal release of ankyloglossia: A randomized trial. *Pediatrics, 128*(2), 280-288. https://www.ncbi.nlm.nih.gov/pubmed/21768318

Chitkara, D.K., Bredenoord, A.J., Wang, M., Rucker, M.J., & Talley, N.J. (2005). Aerophagia in children:

144

Characterization of a functional gastrointestinal disorder. *Neurogastroenterololgy & Motility, 17*(4), 518-522.

Courtiol, J. (2011). *The cause and treatment of infant reflux.* www.coliccalm.com/ baby_infant_newborn_articles/acid-reflux.htm

Fernando, C. (1998). *Tongue-tie: From confusion to clarity.* Sydney, Australia: Tandem Publications.

Kotlow, L. (2004a). Oral diagnosis of abnormal frenum attachments in neonates and infants: Evaluation and treatment of the maxillary and lingual frenum using the Erbium: YAG Laser. *Journal of Pediatric Dental Care, 10*(3), 11-14.

Kotlow, L. (2004b). Oral diagnosis of abnormal frenum attachments in neonates and infants. *Journal of Pediatric Dental Care, 10*(3), 26-28.

Kotlow, L. (2011). Diagnosis and treatment of ankylosis and ties maxillary fraenum in infants using Er:YAG and 1064 Diode lasers. *European Archives of Pediatric Dentistry, 12*(2), 106-112.

Kotlow, L. (2010). The influence of the maxillary frenum on the development and pattern of dental caries on anterior teeth in breastfeeding infants: Prevention, diagnosis and treatment. *Journal of Human Lactation, 26(3), 304-308.*

Li, R., Fein, S.B., Chen, J., & Grummer-Strawn, L. (2008). Why mothers stop breastfeeding: Mothers' self-reported reasons for stopping during the 1st year. *Pediatrics, 122,* 69-76.

Loening-Baucke, V. (2000). Aerophagia as causes of gaseous abdominal distention in a toddler. *Journal of Pediatric Gastroenterology & Nutrition, 32*(2), 204-207.

LAM method of birth control
http://www.waba.org.my/resources/lam/

Campino C, Torres C, Rioseco A, Poblete A, Pugin E, Valdes V, Catalan S,Belmar C, Seron-Ferre M. Plasma prolactin/oestradiol ratio at 38 weeks gestation predicts the duration of lactational amenorrhoea. Hum Reprod. 2001 Dec;16(12):2540-5. "At 38 weeks gestation, the ratio PRL/oestradiol identified all individual women according to the subsequent duration of their lactational amenorrhoea, suggesting that duration of lactational amenorrhoea is conditioned during pregnancy."

Ellison, PT. Breastfeeding, Fertility, and Maternal Condition. In: Stuart-Macadam P, Dettwyler KA, ed. Breastfeeding: Biocultural Perspectives. Hawthorne, NY: Aldine de Gruyter, 1995:305-345.

Eslami SS, Gray RH, Apelo R, Ramos R. The reliability of menses to indicate the return of ovulation in breastfeeding women in Manila, The Philippines. Stud Fam Plann. 1990 Sep-Oct;21(5):243-50.

Gray RH, Campbell OM, Apelo R, Eslami SS, Zacur H, Ramos RM, Gehret JC, Labbok MH. Risk of ovulation during lactation. Lancet. 1990 Jan 6;335(8680):25-9.

Howie PW, McNeilly AS, Houston MJ, Cook A, Boyle H. Fertility after childbirth: infant feeding patterns, basal PRL levels and post-partum ovulation. Clin Endocrinol (Oxf). 1982 Oct;17(4):315-22.

Several papers and discussions on fertility and breastfeeding from The United Nations University Press *Food and Nutrition Bulletin* Volume 17, Number 4, December 1996.

Why to avoid giving bottles until your baby is six weeks old https://massbreastfeeding.org/wp-content/uploads/2013/05/Just-One-Bottle-2014.pdf

Dairy and allergic issues in breastfed babies

https://www.askdrsears.com/topics/health-concerns/fussy-baby/coping-with-colic Coping with Colic by Dr. Bill and Martha Sears. Includes information on tracking down the hidden causes of colic. Tracking Down Food Allergies by Dr. Bill and Martha Sears.

Sicherer SH. Clinical aspects of gastrointestinal food allergy in childhood. Pediatrics. 2003 Jun;111(6 Pt 3):1609-16.
https://www.ncbi.nlm.nih.gov/pubmed/12777600

ABM Clinical Protocol #24: Allergic Proctocolitis in the Exclusively Breastfed Infant
The Academy of Breastfeeding Medicine
https://abm.memberclicks.net/assets/DOCUMENTS/PROTOCOLS/24-allergic-proctocolitis-protocol-english.pdf

Whole Foods For the Whole Family Cookbook edited by Roberta Bishop Johnson, published by La Leche League International, ISBN 0912500433. This book has a large number of dairy-, egg-, and (to a lesser extent) wheat-free recipes.